DON'T DO SOMETHING, JUST STAND THERE

A Primer for Evidence-Based Practice

Frank Cohen

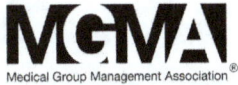

DON'T DO SOMETHING, JUST STAND THERE

A Primer for Evidence-Based Practice

Frank Cohen

Medical Group Management Association© (MGMA©) publications are intended to provide current and accurate information and are designed to assist readers in becoming more familiar with the subject matter covered. Such publications are distributed with the understanding that MGMA does not render any legal, accounting, or other professional advice that may be construed as specifically applicable to an individual situation. No representations or warranties are made concerning the application of legal or other principles discussed by the authors to any specific factual situation, nor is any prediction made concerning how any particular judge, government official, or other person will interpret or apply such principles. Specific factual situations should be discussed with professional advisors.

As of press time, the URLs displayed in this book link or refer to existing websites on the internet. MGMA and EGZ Publications are not responsible for, and should not be deemed to endorse or recommend, any website other than their own or any content available on the internet (including without limitation at any website, blog page, information page) that is not created by MGMA or EGZ Publications. The author, similarly, is not responsible for third-party material.

Published By: MGMA
Production / Partner Publisher: EGZ Publications

Library of Congress Cataloging-in-Publication Data: Galley Copy

p. ; cm.
Includes bibliographical references and index.

ISBN: 978-1-56829-675-3
Medicine--Practice. 2. Medical offices--Management.
I. Medical Group Management Association. II. Title.
[DNLM: 1. Practice Management, Medical. W 80]

Item 1013
ISBN: 978-1-56829-675-3

Copyright © 2019 Frank Cohen and the Medical Group Management Association.

All rights reserved. No part of this publication may be reproduced, stored in a retrieval system, or transmitted, in any form or by any means, electronic, mechanical, photocopying, recording, or otherwise, without the prior written permission of the copyright owners.

CPT codes copyright 2019 American Medical Association. All Rights Reserved. CPT is a trademark of the AMA. No for schedules, basic units, relative values, or related listings are included in CPT. The AMA assumes no liability for the data contained herein. Applicable FARS/DFARS restrictions apply to government use.

Published in Centennial, Colorado
Medical Group Management Association

Printed in the United States of America   10 9 8 7 6 5 4 3 2 1

Contents

Foreword	vii
Preface	xi
Introduction	xxi
Chapter 1　Abracadabra	1
Optical Illusions and Sleight of Evidence-Based	1
Chapter 2　Understanding Management	7
About the Evidence	10
Chapter 3　Paper or Plastic?	13
A Seven Step Decision-Making Process	16
The Three Levels of Decision Making	23
Decision Theory	28
Asymmetry of Information	35
The Law of Diminishing Returns	37
Rational Decision Making	38
Simple vs. Complex Systems	39
Rational Decision Theory	41
Game Theory	48
To Sum Up . . .	57
Chapter 4　It's All About the Evidence	61

Chapter 5 Basic Statistics for the Healthcare Manager	69
Measures of Position and Central Tendency	69
Variance	75
Distributions	80
Error and Confidence Interval	85
Precision	92
Chapter 6 Predicting like a Pro	93
Linear Decomposition	99
Prediction by Analogy	100
Extrapolation Method	101
Trend Analysis	103
Scenario Method	104
The Fermi Method (Dimensional Analysis)	105
Diversity Prediction Theorem	108
Chapter 7 Problem Solving	111
The Monty Hall Problem	113
The Birthday Paradox	116
The Census Problem	118
Chapter 8 Process Improvement as a Composite Model	123
In Closing	*133*
Reference Notes and Resources	*137*
Glossary	*143*
About the Author	*151*

Foreword

By Nate Moore

Frank Cohen is a treasure for the MGMA community.

If you have had the pleasure of hearing Frank speak, the tone of this book will be familiar to you. Even though Frank reads widely across fields the rest of us mere mortals struggle to pronounce, he brings that knowledge down to a level that can be applied and understood. When I look for sessions to attend at an MGMA conference, my first selection criteria is not topics, but presenters. Many of you will remember Frank's presentations in years past. Frank will often turn over his name tag on his lanyard, introduce "Frank Cohen" in the third person, then reverse the name tag saying, "Hi, I'm Frank Cohen." Frank has a habit of showing a lot of funny videos to attendees to break up some fairly technical presentations. I remember a video that showed two people on an escalator in an office building. When the escalator suddenly broke down, the people called for assistance and waited on the escalator for help to arrive. They kept calling and kept waiting, but never made the decision to simply walk up the stalled escalator to freedom.

Making better decisions is the subject of Frank's new book, *Don't Do Something, Stand There!* The providers we serve are trained to make clinical decisions based on data, and we should do the same on the business side. As Frank describes decision-making theory, how to evaluate data, and describes the fundamentals of statistical analysis, take the time to relate his examples directly to issues in your practice. Gathering relevant data may take time. Sometimes the data exists in a canned report, but more often the data might need to be manually entered, or entered consistently, before you can analyze it. You might need IT help to get that data out of your system into a tool for analysis. It may take more time to analyze alternatives, to formulate plans for action, to act, and to evaluate results.

My encouragement is twofold: take the time, but do not expect the time to take forever. Frank describes decision-making processes that include "Ready, ready, ready, ready...", "Ready, aim, ready, aim, ready, aim...," and "Fire, fire, fire, fire, fire...."Getting better data out of your systems to make better decisions should not leave you stuck at "Ready."Impatiently firing without data will not help either. My experience is that practices who get the data they need have returns on that investment faster and higher than they initially expect.

Do not wait until your information is perfect before firing. Frank describes tools and methods to deal with uncertainty and to predict future outcomes. If the best data you have is that there will be five no shows in the North location tomorrow, experiment with that data and act. That may mean you double-book appointments. More data may tell you that the clinic is more successful adding the double-book appointment at 10:00 a.m. instead of 2:00 p.m. More data may instead tell you that your effort is better spent getting three of those five no shows to keep their appointment than it is to fill the slots with other patients. Even more data may tell you the most efficient way to get those patients to show up or ways to adjust provider templates. The process Frank describes is an iterative one, but the rewards are well worth the effort.

Medical practice managers who understand how to use data, how to describe data (yes, even a little statistics), and how to be appropriately skeptical about data will be much more likely to thrive in the ambiguity of today's competitive healthcare environment. Frank will give you the tools you need to start or continue down that road.

Frank's mantra is, "We will no longer make decisions without data." If you and your practice want to make better decisions, your mantra should be, "We will no longer make decisions without applying principles in this book." The book should be required reading for anyone making decisions in the uncertainty of today's healthcare environment.

Preface

My name is Frank Cohen, and I am a computational statistician. I wasn't always a computational statistician, but I have always been a mathematician; at least I knew that was what I was going to be since I was ten years old. My teacher, Mrs. Tennenhouse, made sure that she made math fun and my imagination and obsession was captured that first day. Every day since then has simply been an expansion of that obsession, and today, it is the fulfillment of everything I have ever dreamed it could be.

I have always wondered what it was that made some people love math and others hate it, because it does seem to be a binary relationship. I am to a degree convinced that much of the foundation for those who love math was exposure to great math teachers, and those who don't love math had not-so-great teachers. But I also recognize that at least some of our ability to capture the fascination and imagination that mathematics has to offer has to do with our brain. What, you might ask, does this have to do with a book on evidence-based practice? That is a great question. The answer is that mathematics is based in logic and requires critical thinking, and critical thinking is the big precursor to evidence-based practice. So, if I am going to be able to tell this amazing story, I need to start from the beginning, and that beginning is centered on the human brain.

I will start by saying that I believe the word 'awesome' is overused in our society. A friend of mine once exclaimed: "It would be awesome if I could get a date with Jennifer Lopez." My response was: "It would be statistically impossible, not awesome." Imagining an intelligent design of the universe is awesome. The fact that everything in nature with a spiral follows the Fibonacci sequence is awesome. The fact that water expands when it both boils and freezes is awesome. And the human brain is awesome. In fact, in my opinion, the brain, whether human or not, is the most awesome thing ever!

Corvids, which are birds that include crows, ravens, and rooks, have a brain that could fit in a thimble, yet they are capable of amazing feats. Crows have great problem-solving skills and are even capable of performing sequential tasks to solve problems. In one of Aesop's tales, "The Crow and the Pitcher," the story tells of a crow that came across a tall pitcher that had only a few inches of water at the bottom. Hard as he might try, the crow could not get his head and neck far enough into the narrow opening to reach the water to drink. The fable goes on like this: "Then an idea came to him. Picking up some small pebbles, he dropped them into the pitcher, one by one. With each pebble, the water rose a little higher until at last it was near enough so he could drink."

In a study by Christopher Bird and Nathan Emery published online in the August 6, 2009, edition of the journal *Current Biology*, the authors reported that they were able to get rooks to do just what Aesop's tale said they could. They placed a floating worm in some water at the bottom of a long tube, and the rooks used the pebbles to raise the water level to a point where they were able to reach the worm. The study authors constructed a box with an upper section that formed a small tube: too small for the rooks to fit through. In the bottom of the box, they placed a small bucket with some food in it. At the top of the tube, they placed a straight piece of wire. The rook used the wire to try to retrieve the bucket and, eventually, made a bend in the bottom of the wire to create a hook. From there, they were able to hook the bucket and bring it to the surface.

In a book called *Gifts of the Crow: How Perception, Emotion, and Thought Allow Smart Birds to Behave Like Humans* (2012), by John Marzluff and Tony Angell, the authors concluded that crows can remember faces (a function of the hippocampus) for at least a decade. In the study, a researcher wearing a mask would come into courtyard and harass a bunch of crows. In response, the crows would also harass the researcher. Each subsequent time the researcher walked into the courtyard with the mask, even though he was not harassing the crows, they would harass him. When he walked out without the mask, the crows ignored him. Then he gave the mask to a colleague, and when that colleague wore the mask into the courtyard, he was immediately harassed by the crows. And all this in a bird's brain. Imagine how awesome is the human brain!

The average adult brain has nearly 100 billion neurons, or specialized brain cells. In fact, according to a study published in the April 2009 edition of the *Journal of Comparative Neurology*, the average human brain has 86.1 billion neurons plus or minus 8.1 billion. That's a lot of cells, and I think that we often overlook just how many of anything make up a billion. For example, if you were to count to a million, skipping meals and sleep, it would take you 11.5 non-stop days. But a billion, that's a whole different story. To count to a billion would take you approximately 33 years, so to count all the neurons in the human brain would take 2,481 years. This certainly qualifies as awesome! Each of those 86.1 billion neurons can connect to thousands, if not tens-of-thousands of other neurons and, even though there is a bit of disagreement over the total number of possible connections, most will agree that it is at least 100 trillion. That's more connections in the human brain than there are stars in the universe. Come on, that's truly awesome.

The brain is broken up into a series of *lobes*: large sections of the brain that contain similar type neurons and perform some specific tasks. These areas are the occipital lobe, the parietal lobe, the temporal lobe, the cerebellum, and the frontal lobe. The *occipital lobe*, which is located at the back of the brain, is responsible for processing visual information from the eyes. But not just vision, like seeing things, but when connected to other parts of the brain, seeing things dimensionally. The ability to do geometry is associated with visual-spatial representations, which is accomplished through connections between the occipital lobe and the parietal lobe. The *parietal lobe* processes sensory information, like sounds and smell and touch. It also works to help interpret visual information, process language, and some areas of mathematics. The *temporal lobe* processes much of our hearing and auditory stimuli, while the *cerebellum* controls movement and balance. Athletes have really high-functioning cerebellums. But what really separates us from lower forms of life, specifically as it pertains to critical thinking, is the *frontal lobe*. This is the portion of the brain that sits right behind our forehead, and in the average person, the frontal lobe accounts for between 33% and 38% of the total brain. The closest mammal to us that has anything like it is the Rhesus monkey, whose frontal lobe accounts for 17%, or about half of that in the human brain. The frontal lobe of a dog's brain makes up about 7.5% of total brain volume, while for a cat, it is around 3%.

Again, it is fair to ask why this is important and why it is part of a book on evidence-based practice. The answer is: it is the frontal lobe of the brain where critical thinking originates, and without critical thinking, we won't become successful evidence-based practitioners. The frontal lobe itself is divided into different cortices. The *prefrontal cortex* manages complex cognitive processes, such as memory, planning, reasoning, and problem-solving, all critical skills for the evidence-based practitioner. But since this is not a book on the neurophysiology of the brain, we are going to stay a little higher level in the upcoming discussion. Just remember that I am going to be generalizing on cortical components but not on functional processes. From the most basic perspective, the frontal lobe is the command and control center for the entire brain. While the other lobes can function independently of the frontal lobe, it is the frontal lobe that mediates those functions. For example, movement activates frontal lobe activity, even though the frontal lobe is not responsible for that movement. Walking is a function of the cerebellum as well as the parietal lobes, but the frontal lobe mediates that activity. In a healthy brain, it prevents us from walking into traffic or into a dangerous situation.

We can speak, *per se*, without interacting with the frontal lobe because understanding words and concepts occurs in the *angular gyrus* and a section called *Wernicke's area,* and the motor skills for speech occur in the temporal lobe. But there is an area in the frontal lobe that mediates our language; in essence, it allows us to make sense of what we are saying. It also controls the executive function of speech, assessing things like "Is what I am about to say appropriate?" Have you ever said anything and then and instant later wish you could take it back? Or how about someone who seems to put their mouth in gear before their brain is engaged? These can be symptoms of a compromised frontal lobe.

The frontal lobes are involved in motor function, problem solving, spontaneity, memory, language, initiation, judgment, impulse control, and social and sexual behavior. But perhaps of greatest importance, at least for the purpose of this book, the frontal lobe is the center for reasoning, planning, and problem solving, all of which determine the quality of the decisions we make. Evidence-based practice, whether in medicine or administration and management, is all about making good decisions. So, if we follow the logic, in order to be a good evidence-based practitioner, we need to have a healthy frontal lobe. And a healthy frontal lobe is dependent on what we take in with respect to our senses and our diet.

Check this out: you are at a conference and you see someone. Remember, visual processing is performed by the occipital lobe. It is interpreting what your eyes are seeing. Then, using your temporal lobe, you recognize the person's face. The hippocampus, which is part of the *limbic system*, kicks in, and you remember that this person insulted you a few years ago at a party. Suddenly, thanks to the *amygdala*, you start to get angry. In this scenario, probably the only thing that would prevent you from going up to that person and starting a fight is the frontal lobe, because it is the mediator of those emotions.

One of my favorite stories is about a man by the name of Phineas Gage. He was a blasting foreman for an American railroad company. Back in the mid 1800's, Phineas was working on laying railroad tracks for the Rutland & Burlington Railroad outside of Cavendish, Vermont. It was a rocky area, and in order to get the track through, workers often had to set blast charges to blow up rocks. The process involved drilling a deep hole into an outcrop of rocks, putting powder in the hole and then filling it the rest of the way with sand. Then, a worker would take a tamping iron, which weighed about 20 pounds, and pack the sand down to control and focus the blast. On September 13, 1848, at around 4:30 p.m., while tamping one of the holes, an explosion occurred and the tamping rod blew out of the hole, passing through Phineas' jaw, behind his left eye and exiting out the front of his skull. Within just a few minutes, Phineas was up and talking. Shortly thereafter, he was hospitalized and underwent surgery and treatment for his injuries.

Amazingly, within six months of his injury, Phineas returned to work. But by all accounts, he was no longer the same man. Before the injury, Phineas was greatly liked and respected by his men. He was considered to have been intelligent, personable, and a tough but very fair boss. But after the injury, his personality completely changed. He became angry and irritated at the drop of a hat. Due to the change in his behavior, he was not welcome to return to his previous position, even though his mental acuity and physical prowess appeared unimpaired. Why the change? The injury had all but destroyed the frontal lobe of his brain. His doctor noted that immediately after his injury, Phineas was "gross, profane, coarse and vulgar, to such a degree that his society was intolerable to decent people."

You don't need to have traumatic injury to compromise your frontal lobe. Alcohol impacts the frontal lobe before it impacts any other part of the brain. If you were to have just one drink, you would likely still be able to pass a sobriety test: walking a straight line (the cerebellum and occipital lobe), recite the alphabet (temporal lobe), touch your fingers to your nose, etc. But at half of the legal drinking limit of only 0.04%, your chances of being involved in a crash is four times higher than if you hadn't had any alcohol at all. At the legal limit of 0.08%, most people could still pass a sobriety test but would have a twelve-fold chance of being involved in a crash. Why is that, particularly if the motor and visual cortices are operating properly? It's because our judgment, which is encased in our critical thinking ability, is compromised.

Does this mean that it requires critical thinking to operate a car? I don't think so. Driving a car is based mostly on heuristics, or rule sets. For example, my 12-year-old grandson can drive my Yamaha

Rhino around my property with a great deal of success. He understands the rules: press on the gas and it goes faster, press on the brake and it slows down. Turn the wheel to the left and the Rhino goes left, turn the wheel to the right and the Rhino goes right. But the first time he took a corner a bit too fast, without a fully developed frontal lobe and lacking the experience of a more seasoned driver, he hit a tree. This was because he lacked the judgment to think outside of the rule set, or more colloquially, outside the box. How long does it take the frontal lobe to fully develop? The consensus is around 30 years, so if you are under 30 and have made some bad decisions, don't be so hard on yourself; we are all in the same boat.

Driving a car, then, doesn't necessarily require critical thinking. But driving a car in anything other than average conditions might require critical thinking. Going down the highway on a sunny day? Heuristics. Avoiding hitting a deer that jumps out from the ditch? Critical thinking. I remember the hysterics when Lady Di was killed in a car crash back in 1997. Her driver was trying to avoid the paparazzi that were following her when they entered a tunnel. Trying to navigate a turn in a dark tunnel at high speeds, the car crashed, and the former Princess of Wales died from her injuries. There was a lot of speculation that followed, including that her driver, Henri Paul was drunk, and according to the autopsy report, that was true. It should also be noted that Henri Paul had special driving training and skills but alcohol affects the frontal lobe before any other part of the brain, so while he was still able to drive the vehicle from a purely heuristic point of view, his reasoning and judgment were compromised, causing him to approach the curve at a speed (121 mph) that was simply faster than the vehicle was able to navigate.

How about an airplane? Does flying an airplane require critical thinking? Again, I don't think so. I have a friend who is a pilot, and I went flying with him a few times. After the third flight, I was able to take off, fly, and the land the airplane successfully. This is based on heuristics, muscle memory, a basic ability to learn, and physical capabilities that originate from other areas of the brain. But what does require critical thinking is when the plane encounters bad weather or a malfunction or high winds on landing. Judgment and reasoning, thinking outside the box, can mean the difference between life and death in more challenging situations.

Here's an example. Back in 2009, AirFrance flight 447 was flying between Rio de Janeiro, Brazil and Paris, France. It was controlled by a pilot and two co-pilots. At some point in the flight, ice had formed in the pitot tubes, which are responsible for measuring how fast the plane is flying. As a result, the autopilot disengaged, which caused the engines' auto-thrust systems to disengage as well. Due to turbulence, and possibly improper manual control of the plane, the airspeed indicator showed that the plane was flying too fast. What's the best way for the pilots to slow down a plane? It's for them to push the stick forward and point the nose of the plane up to the sky. The pilots did that, but when they did, they realized that the plane was losing altitude too quickly. The way to solve that problem is to point the nose down, but by the time they realized what was happening (they had gone into a tail stall), they did not have enough altitude left. They crashed into the Atlantic Ocean, killing everyone aboard.

Eventually, the recovery of the black boxes allowed investigators to follow those terrifying last seven-and-a-half minutes, both with a record of the plane's movements and instrument readings, as well as the conversation between the pilot and the copilots. As it turns out, they did everything they should have done based on the information they were getting from the computer. In essence, they did it by the book. But they still crashed. Why? There are seven instruments that a pilot relies upon to fly a plane at night or in really bad weather. This is called IFR, or *instrument flight rating* as opposed to VFR, which stands for *visual flight rating*. The latter is what occurs during clear weather and high visibility conditions. Those pilots had seven-and-a-half minutes to figure out which instrument was defective, and they couldn't do it. They followed the manual to the T, but it wasn't enough because the manual didn't help them to figure out which instrument was bad. In the end, they missed it, and the consequences were tragic to say the least.

It came down to the pilots' ability to engage in critical thinking; to think outside the box. They needed to disregard the heuristics and engage all the frontal lobe had to offer, using complex reasoning skills to solve a problem that meant the difference between life and death. Just look at the events that unfolded when Captain Sullenberger, piloting US Airways flight 1549, had to respond to an emergency on January 15, 2009. It had just taken off from LaGuardia airport in New Jersey when both engines were struck by Canada geese and subsequently disabled. Captain Sullenberger and his copilot had only a few moments to find a solution to a problem for which there was no prior case study nor that was within the capability of the plane's computer system. And they did it, landing safely on the Hudson River, saving every passenger and crew member on board. According to Captain Sullenberger, "Within two and a half seconds, I had begun to take the first two remedial actions by memory. I turned on the engine ignition and started the aircraft's auxiliary power unit." Thinking outside the box, exercising complex decision-making and problem-solving skills resulted in a positive outcome from a seemingly impossible decision and all this as a result of the frontal lobe of the brain. Awesome!

To be a critical thinker, you don't need to be successful at evidence-based practice, but to be successful at evidence-based practice, you need to be a critical thinker. We can extend these examples to nearly every area of life, but particularly when we need to make split-second decisions that are not based on solely experience. In those situations, it is our critical thinking skills that determine the difference between success and failure.

Take, for example, how a surgeon thinks. Imagine a surgeon doing something like removing someone's appendix. Let's assume that this surgeon has done these many times. For the most part, the ability to complete this type of a procedure successfully is based on heuristics. There are a certain set of rules that the surgeon will almost always follow for these types of procedures. Basic processes like proper scrubbing and proper preparation of the area are standardized and a matter of habit. Whether the procedure is performed open or scoped will determine the rules for how the skin it cut, how the devices are used, how to deal with bleeding, and how to avoid damaging surrounding structure. But say something happens that is both unexpected, and a situation that the surgeon hasn't experienced before. The difference between a positive and negative outcome, maybe the life or death of a patient, will depend on how well that surgeon can create (imagine, formulate, reason) a solution for a situation that s/he has never encountered before.

Let's not be fooled by this example: surgeons are highly trained and intelligent people. They go through four years of undergraduate school, four years of medical school, residencies, internships, more training, more residencies and on and on it goes. Doctors are perhaps the most highly trained and skilled individuals one may ever encounter. And while intelligence is a result of high frontal lobe function, critical thinking is an even higher function of the frontal lobe. It would be great if we could simulate every possible scenario in life, but the fact is, we just can't. So doing everything we can (diet and exercise, avoiding alcohol and caffeine, to controlling what enters the brain through our other senses) just about guarantee that anyone (more like everyone) can experience the benefits of critical thinking that will result in a highly functional and successful evidence-based practitioner. I hope this book is a useful tool for you to further your progress along this journey.

Introduction

The story goes that there was this scientist who was interested in studying the impact of different environmental conditions on earthworms. So, he set up an experiment where he took four beakers and in each of the four beakers established some different environmental condition. In the first beaker, he put some ethanol from a popular whiskey. In the second beaker, he put chocolate syrup. He filled the third beaker with cigarette smoke, and in the fourth beaker, he put fresh dirt. Then he placed an earthworm in each of the four beakers and went home. The next morning when he came in, he observed that the earthworm in beaker one, filled with whiskey, was dead. The worm in the beaker of chocolate syrup was also dead, as was the worm that was in the beaker filled with cigarette smoke. In the fourth beaker, which contained fresh dirt, the earthworm was alive and well. So, what conclusion do you think the scientists came up with based on the results of the study? Go ahead, I'll wait . . . Their conclusion was this: if you drink, smoke, and eat chocolate, you won't get worms.

Now I know that this is a joke. But what it describes is not far from how scientists draw conclusions from within their studies about their experiments. In fact, within the scientific community, we are in a bit of a crisis of integrity, most often referred to as a crisis of replication. On February 22, 2017, the BBC published an article online entitled "Most of Scientists Can't Replicate Studies by Their Peers." At face value, that's pretty scary, because at the heart of scientific study is the ability to replicate the results of a scientific experiment. In May 2016, *Nature* magazine published the results of a survey they conducted on reproducibility amongst 1,576 researchers. The results? More than 70% of the researchers who responded stated that they have tried and failed to reproduce another scientist's experiment and just over half said they had failed to reproduce their own experiments.

A couple of years ago, I attended the Joint Statistical Meetings of the American Statistical Association, and one of the primary speakers addressed this issue. Pretty much everyone I spoke with at that meeting agreed that it was in fact a crisis. The reasons that this is occurring are broad and alarming. In academic institutions, it's because of pressure placed upon instructors to publish, which is very important for obtaining a full professorship. In the private sector, much of it has to do with money. There is a tremendous amount of competition for grants and for granted dollars. Whatever the reason, the impact is felt broadly across all industries. In this book, where we discuss critical thinking, much of the decision-making process must be based upon evidence. What is evidence? In general, it is that which tends to prove or disprove something. When making decisions, evidence provides a foundation for our conclusions. Perhaps, then, as important as evidence is in and of itself, it is just as important to have a foundational understanding of data analytics and scientific study. I can assure you that those are topics this book will cover.

Sir Isaiah Berlin's "The Hedgehog and the Fox"

But first, a story by one of my favorite philosophers, Sir Isaiah Berlin. It is from an essay entitled "The Hedgehog and the Fox: An Essay on Tolstoy's View of History."

> A fox and a hedgehog were strolling through a country path. Periodically, they were threatened by hungry wolves. The fox—being blessed with smarts, speed and agility — would lead the packs of wolves on a wild chase through the fields, up and down trees, and over hill and dale. Eventually the fox would return to the path, breathless but having lost the wolves, and continue walking. The hedgehog, being endowed with a coat of spikes, simply hunkered down on its haunches

when menaced by the wolves and fended them off without moving. When they gave up, he would return to his stroll unperturbed.

This essay addresses two primary lenses that people use to see the world and to define their ideas. The hedgehog sees the world through the lens of a single defining idea. This reminds me of the heuristic that says if the only tool you have is a hammer then pretty soon everything starts to look like a nail. In his essay, Berlin wrote, "Hedgehogs have the keen ability to focus and drive along a single path." Jim Collins, author of the book *Good to Great*, says,

> Those who built the good-to-great companies were, to one degree or another, hedgehogs. They used their hedgehog nature to drive toward what we came to call a Hedgehog Concept for their companies. Those who led the comparison companies tended to be foxes, never gaining the clarifying advantage of a Hedgehog Concept, being instead scattered, diffused, and inconsistent.

The hedgehog has a highly focused and narrow view, not only of the world, but of solutions to problems and interpretations of evidence. On the other hand, the fox draws on a wide variety of experiences, and sees the world through more of a prism than a single lens. For the fox, distilling the world to just a single idea is impossible. Isaiah Berlin wrote, "Foxes are complex thinkers who account for a variety of circumstances and experiences."

From a leadership perspective, whether a person follows the direction of a hedgehog or a fox can determine their success or failure within specified work cultures and environments. But for the purposes of this book, we are talking about their thought processes as they pertain to critical thinking. Hedgehogs are often subject to confirmation bias. They see the world through a selective lens, and it tends to filter out those ideas and data and evidence that do not conform to those ideas or that belief system. As much as I would like to think that I have tendencies of the fox, I am much more like the hedgehog. I am a mathematician. In fact, I focus on computational mathematics, which relies upon advanced and applied statistics and predictive modeling and machine learning to solve problems. So, when I get together with people who tend to look at the world through a broader base of heuristics, meaning those people who rely upon nonlogical approaches to problem-solving or decision-making, I can't relate. I believe you can measure anything. If it's physically observable within the universe, it is measurable using logic and models.

I was once advising a physician to help him determine whether he was going to continue in private practice or go to work for the local hospital as an employee. As we talked, he made the comment, "You can't measure happiness." I disagree. In fact, for everyone I've ever met, happiness is absolutely an observable emotion. So, I asked him what makes him happy. "Well," he said, "having more free time would make me happy." Next, I asked him how much free time he would need to be happy, and he gave me a number. That was a measurement. He also talked about revenue. He said he needed to earn a certain amount of money to be happy. Can we measure revenue? Of course. He also talked about not having to be on call all the time. I asked him to define "all the time," and he gave me the number of days per month that would be the limit for him. Can we measure days? Of course, we can. By the time this discussion was complete, I was able to quantify those aspects of his life that defined happiness for him in this situation.

Are you a fox or a hedgehog? The answer will help you to determine your strengths and weaknesses as an evidence-based manager. Both worldviews are capable of critical thinking and both play a vital role in our management philosophies. If nothing else, what it should tell us is that we should always consider the importance of inclusion and diversity when faced with complex problems. Remember, our goal is to increase the probability that our management decisions will result in a positive outcome.

Malcom Gladwell is one of my favorite authors. In 2005, he published a book called *Blink: The Power of Thinking Without Thinking*. In general, Gladwell focuses on something called "thin-slicing," which is the ability to use limited (or thin slices) of information within a narrowly focused event to come to some conclusion or result. While he gets into some detail regarding unconscious and subconscious thought, my take was that he was really addressing our ability to use intuition (hence the "without thinking" part) to make decisions or draw conclusions.

While I am a fan of intuition, I disagree that we should rely upon it to make decisions or come to conclusions, particularly in critical situations. Think back to the story of the scientists and the worms. How did that work out?

I believe that intuition is useful to guide study design. We can use subconscious and unconscious experiences that we have had to point us in the right direction.

It's Okay to Be Lucky When You're Lucky

My dad used to say, "It's okay to be lucky when you're lucky," and that's fine in noncritical situations. But most of us who are engaged in managing healthcare organizations are involved in day-to-day decisions that have an elevated level of criticality. In those cases, intuition and anecdote can be more dangerous than they are helpful.

I heard this great joke one time. A guy tells a story where he was out on a camping trip with a friend of his. As they were sitting around the fire, his friend gets bit on the leg by snake. So, the comedian takes out his smart phone and takes a picture of the snake and walks out of the campsite to get a signal, where he calls a local hospital. They ask him to forward a picture of the snake, and when he does, they tell him that this is a coral snake and that it contains a neurotoxin. Unless his friend gets an antidote, he's going to die. So, he goes back to the campsite, and he starts telling his friend funny stories. Several hours later, his friend dies. After the paramedics come and take his friend away, he concluded that had he known the difference between "anecdote" and "antidote," his friend would still be alive. What we want here is an antidote. We want solutions to problems that are based on logic, evidence, and the use of analytics. So, let's start by talking about the evidence.

Why should we even rely upon evidence? Why not upon intuition or anecdote?

Think of the times you have seen a problem or situation that looks like another problem or situation, and so, you apply the same problem-solving techniques to this situation, but it doesn't work? I know that this has happened to me more times than I care to admit. It worked before so why not this time? Anecdote looks at a broad spectrum of issues. It deals with the 30,000-foot view, and if you've ever studied fractals, you know that it's the details that drive the models.

Can we trust what we see and what we hear? My opinion is no.

It is strange to me how often people defend their positions by saying, "Oh, I read it on the internet." They treat the internet as some final authority of truth, honesty, and integrity. I mean, look at the technology that we have today and our ability to edit and manipulate digital images (still photos or videos). Any home computer can create photos and videos that look legitimate but are actually fundamentally different from what really occurred.

Believe Nothing You Hear, and Only One-Half That You See

In the short story "The System of Dr. Tarr and Professor Fether," by Edgar Allan Poe, the head of a mental institution states the following: "'You are young yet, my friend,' replied my host, 'but the time will arrive when you will learn to judge for yourself of what is going on in the world, without trusting to the gossip of others. *Believe nothing you hear, and only one-half that you see* (emphasis added).'" This saying has since been repeated *ad nauseum* in application to everything from the California Gold Rush (1848-1855) to the Norman Whitfield and Barrett Strong song "I Heard it through the Grapevine" released by Motown records in September 1967, produced by Whitfield, and featuring the renowned Gladys Knight & the Pips. The crux is that our brains are fallible and subject to interpretation and estimation that render them untrustworthy. In fact, our brains construct our reality based on only a small portion of the information (data or evidence) available.

Introduction

In a jury trial, which is the epitome of the evidence-based critical thought process, no one is ever 100% certain of anything. In the legal system, there are two standards of proof that must be met to determine the outcome of a case. "Preponderance of the evidence" is found in civil cases and is the lower of the two. Here, the person bringing a suit or charge must prove that there is a greater than 50% likelihood that their claim is true; that the defendant did wrong or caused damage. In a criminal case, there is a much higher burden of proof: "beyond a reasonable doubt." While there isn't a specific probability value attached to this standard, I have worked with attorneys that state the likelihood that the defendant committed the crime is upwards or greater than 95%.

In either of these standards, there really isn't any way to measure the exact probability. It is difficult to say, with certainty, that we are exactly 52% certain or 71% certain; it is more a 'feeling' that we have regarding the truth. Unless and until we can get inside the head of the defendant and see and experience what they experienced, getting to 100% is pretty much impossible. That means that, within our system of justice, we sometimes acquit guilty people and find innocent people guilty. This equitably describes the reliability of the human brain. So, I will ask the question again; do we believe what we see, or do we see what we believe, or do we see what we want to see?

Let's examine what happens when some traumatic event occurs, like a violent crime. In a National Academy of Sciences landmark report on memory and eyewitness identification, they found that eyewitness misidentification was a predominant contributing factor to wrongful convictions. Using DNA testing as a standard, misidentification played at least some role in the reversal of 72% of 318 wrongful convictions. How is that possible? One idea has to do with the difference between recognition and recall, and while I don't want to turn this into a scientific treatise on the brain, I do think that it's important to understand why evidence trumps intuition.

In a 2017 study by the Reysen Group called "The Relationship between the Big 5 Personality Traits and Eyewitness Recognition," which was published in *The Journal of Articles in Support of the Null Hypothesis*, the authors concluded that recognition centers on the judgment of the person or event and whether the stimulus has been viewed before, while recall is solely dependent upon one's memories and may very well be judgment-independent. Although the study goes into depth about how these concepts interact with different memory traits, suffice it to say that the primary problem is still with a high level of eyewitness misidentification.

Look at an example. Let's say that you are in a convenience store and two individuals enter the store with guns blazing, screaming for everyone to get on the ground. Some people are going to focus on the guns. Others are going to focus on the individuals; their size, weight, what they are wearing, etc. When the police show up and start identifying witnesses, those that focused on the gun will likely be able to describe what they looked like with some degree of accuracy, while others will be better at describing the physical characteristics of the perpetrators. The problem is that those who focused on the gun will likely also attempt to describe the physical attributes of the perpetrators and those who focused on the individuals will likely also attempt to describe the weapons. The complete information will likely be quite inaccurate. What's the solution? In many cases, police and investigators will "average" the information obtained from eyewitnesses, and this has proved to be a better solution than relying only upon the information from an individual.

Have you ever wondered how it is that when you blink while driving, you don't end up going off the road? There are several studies that support the idea that blinking helps us to accurately construct a visual scene. Remember, the visual part of the brain functions on some amount less than all the available data, and as such, needs to create (or imagine) the missing or not present data. When you blink, the brain takes the data from prior to blinking and extends or extrapolates that information to the portion of time where the data stream stops, like when your eyes are closed, or you are looking down. And if you don't take your eyes off the road for too long (like when texting), the brain can usually fill in those blanks such that our consciousness doesn't even know that anything was awry. This opens the door to lots of problems with relying upon anecdote rather than antidote for our management decisions and problem resolution. In fact, it opens the way for exploitation of the sort used by magicians, artists, scammers, and phishers.

The Role of Intuition

Not too long ago, I got an email from someone that I know well that started by simply saying, "How are you? I hope all is well with you. I need a favor from you. Please email me back as soon as possible." And I did. I told this person that I would be happy to assist where possible. And here is the email that I received back:

> I am having such a frustrating ordeal right now. I need to make an urgent deposit to a Doctor today, but I'm out of town until Monday. This deposit is for my Sister-in-Law who has an inflamed gall bladder. She's having a surgery today, because her condition now is very serious. I need your assistance, please I need you to help me make this payment, I'll reimburse you once I get back on Monday, I promise! Please let me know if I can count on you...

At first blush, this seemed like a legitimate request and on follow up, I was given instructions to wire the money via Western Union. And I about did, but right before I completed the transaction, I decided to call this person and verify the request. It turns out that her email account had been hacked and the email I received (which, by the way, everyone else in her contact list received) was a scam. In the immortal words of Maxwell Smart, "I missed it by that much." I am willing to bet that many of you reading this are nodding your heads in concurrence as this has also happened to you. What saved me? Well, in the spirit of bias towards my book, evidence. Rather than relying solely upon what I was told (ambiguity effect) and believing it because I know and trust this person (confirmation bias), I took the time, albeit almost too late, to confirm what I believed, and in this case, it turned out that I was (almost) wrong.

This is where intuition comes in strong. Not only is intuition not always a terrible thing, it is proven to save lives, especially when used to stimulate a look at the evidence. Let's look at the development of the Rapid Response Team (RRT). Sometime back in the late 1990's in Australia, we saw the development of what were called call rapid response (or assessment) teams. A short story is that there was a medical unit nurse who, in caring for her patient, notices some changes that were not necessarily evident based on the clinical findings. For example, the patient's temperament changed a bit in a nuanced sort of way. They became a bit more restless and agitated and their speech patterns seemed to change. Again, these were quite nuanced observations, yet there weren't any specific clinical signs to support the nurse's concerns. In any case, she requested the on-call physician, who agreed with the nurse, and after running some stat tests, determined that the patient was, in fact, deteriorating rather quickly. As a result, the medical staff was able to intervene and more than likely saved the patient's life. It is my understanding that this incident generated the creation of the Rapid Response Team (RRT).

We started to see this take hold in the United States starting around the mid 2000's, and today, there are many hospitals that employ and extensively use RRTs. While there are not as many quantitative studies as I would like to see, there are enough to convince me that this is a great idea. Generally, every hospital has a 'code blue' team. This is a multi-disciplinary group of healthcare professionals that respond to patients that are 'coding' or having some cardiovascular failure. The purpose of the RRT is to minimize or at least reduce the number of codes called by identifying the subtle and nuanced signs that often precede a 'code blue' event. To accomplish this, the attending nurse is given a wide latitude and authority to advance a patient to an RRT if s/he feels as though there is 'something wrong' with the patient that may not be supported through traditional clinical evidence. What we are talking about here is intuition, but let's not stop there. This nurse, who is well trained and experienced in caring for his or her patients is, in every sense, a subject matter expert (SME) on recognizing those nuanced changes in patient behavior. If the nurse notices a change and maybe 'can't put a finger on it,' s/he has the authority to call the RRT to come in and check out the patient. There are several studies as well as anecdotal evidence out there to show that the use of the RRT results in a decline in the use of 'code teams' because the patient's condition is addressed before it gets to that level of criticality.

I have seen many articles that focus on the makeup of the team. Some use a physician assistant (PA) as a team leader, and most teams include a respiratory professional, since respiratory problems almost always precede more significant events like heart attacks. Some studies have shown that the use of the RRT has reduced admissions to the ICU from the medical or surgical floors, as problems that may have spiraled out of control were caught in time to treat preemptively. But in the end, it's not really the cross-disciplinary make-up of the team that defines success; it's giving the authority to make critical decisions to those that are in the best position to do act quickly in a crisis. It's important to note that, in the literature, there are many examples of false positives; situations where the nurse called the RRT and it turned out to be nothing, but this is how we learn, grow, and become better at what we do.

In writing software that incorporates machine learning, I often depend upon a feedback loop from the end user. For example, let's say that I analyze a thousand claims and my predictive algorithm picks a bunch that it has determined may have been improperly coded (or billed) for one reason or another. The organization then audits that claim internally and feeds the results back to the application. Let's say in one of those, the auditor finds that the claim was in fact coded and billed properly. The algorithm will then consider this and look to see what was different from this claim (that passed an audit) versus the claim that failed the audit. This is what machine learning is about; the machine learns from its mistakes and tweaks the algorithm so that each time it receives a returned audit the application becomes better and better at its job. The same is true with the RRT example above. In the case of a false positive, the team (which absolutely includes the nurse) should get together and debrief their findings. This feedback loop, rather than impacting an algorithm, impacts the decision-making process of the nurse; to help him or her recognize how a false positive may be generated and ways to avoid it in the future.

While more quantitative studies need to be conducted, there is a general consensus that RRTs save lives and hence we expect to see a continued growth of these and similar programs. This succeeds in these circumstances because it allows intuitive insights from team members to impact the process directly.

CHAPTER 1
Abracadabra

Optical Illusions and Sleight of Hand

Have you ever wondered how magic tricks work to fool us? There are a lot of techniques that magicians can use but, in the end, magic works because we lie to ourselves and then we believe those lies. Let's take a moment to talk about the *red panda effect*. In 1978, a famous and rare red panda escaped from the Rotterdam zoo in the Netherlands. Because, at that time, we didn't have communication services like Twitter or Facebook or Instagram, zoo officials enlisted the assistance of the press to spread the word that the panda had escaped. The word went out via radio and print, and over the next few months, there were nearly two hundred sightings reported. The sad truth is that they found the panda dead shortly after the escape, so the question remains, if they didn't see the red panda, what did these people see? And the answer is really quite simple: they saw what they wanted to see.

In another example, published back in 2001 by the *Journal International des Sciences de la Vigne et du Vin*, Frédéric Brochet, Gil Morrot, and Denis Dubourdieu conducted a sneaky study. In this experiment, Brochet colored a white wine red using a tasteless red food dye. Then, he had fifty-four oenology (wine science) students evaluate the wine. Overwhelmingly, the panel of students described the wine as they would a red wine. With rare exception, they were all fooled, even though they were experts on the science of wine. What was most interesting to me was the conclusion that descriptions of smell are almost entirely based on what we see. Fascinating! Some have used this to conclude that wine tasting is nothing more than a bunch of hooey, but, in reality, it supports what I have been saying all along: our brains are subject to influences that defy truth, fact, and even reality, and as a result, we need to make a conscious effort to look for the truth by understanding and evaluating all the evidence that is available to us.

In art, we see optical illusions all the time. Perhaps the most common is using shading and lines to create a three-dimensional interpretation from a two-dimensional image.

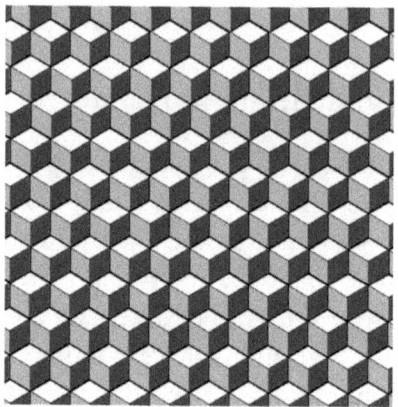

FIGURE 1.1   3D block illusion

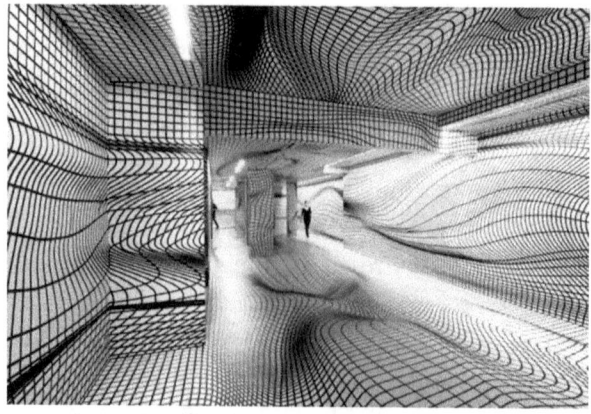

FIGURE 1.2   The wave illusion

The above images are what are known as paradox illusions. These are illusions generated by objects or images that are impossible in real life but look convincing, even when we know that they can't be true. We see this in the Penrose Stairs, a two-dimensional depiction of a three-dimensional staircase created by Lionel Penrose and his son Roger Penrose.

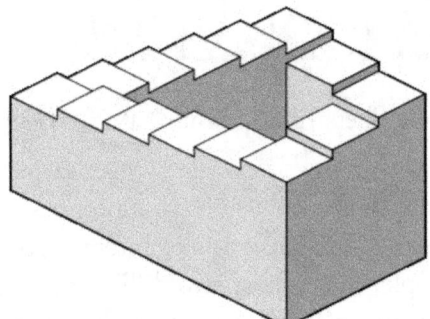

FIGURE 1.3 The Penrose stairs

The illusion in the Penrose Stairs is the concept that a person could continue to climb *ad infinitum* yet never get any higher on the staircase. Another such illusion is a *blivet* called the impossible trident; an image that displays two irreconcilable images at once. Notice that the object on the left appears to have three prongs yet there is a "lost layer" that makes that assumption impossible. We see the same type of illusion with the so-called five-legged elephant. There are five feet, but there are only four legs: an impossible and irreconcilable problem.

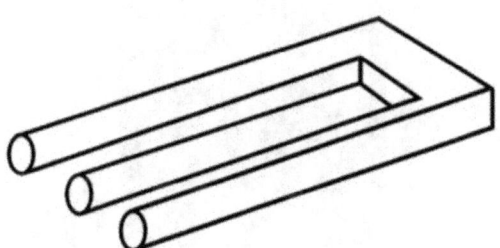

FIGURE 1.4 The impossible trident

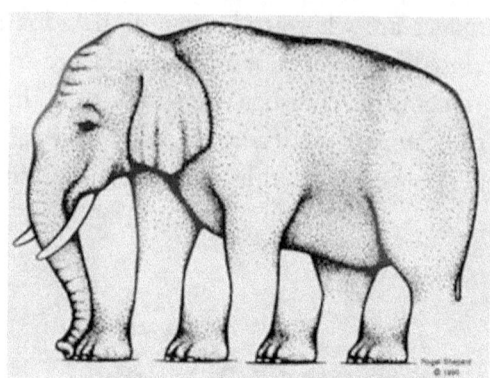

FIGURE 1.5   The Shepard elephant © 1990 Roger Shepard

One of my favorite types of illusions is sometimes called *ambiguous stimuli*. They are illusions that are open to interpretation. Presented to a diverse group of people, they report two different interpretations from the same image. For example, in the picture on below, do you see an old woman or a young woman? Well, if you follow the outline along the left border, you see a nose and a chin of the young woman. If you focus on the image portion near the bottom, you see an older woman's chin, mouth, and then nose.

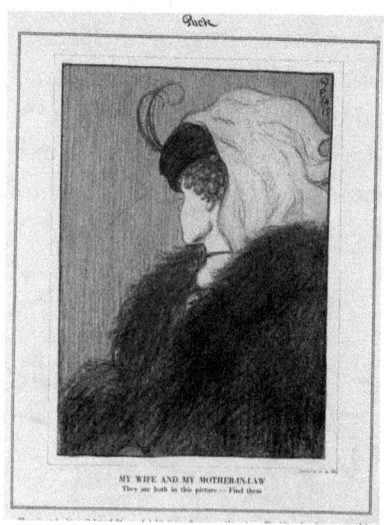

FIGURE 1.6   *My Wife and My Mother-in-Law,* by William Ely Hill

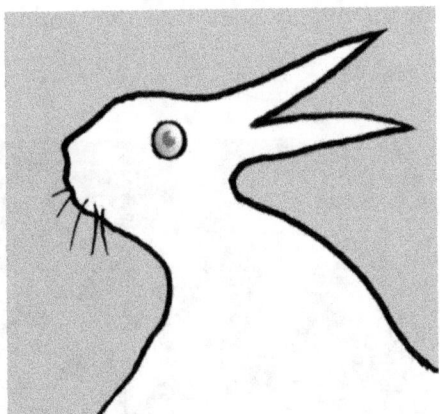

FIGURE 1.7   Duck rabbit illusion

The same is true for the image on the image below. Do you see a rabbit (following the left border) or a duck (following the right border)?

There is even an illusion that deals with the issue of confabulation, which is normally associated with false memories but applies here with the following paragraph:

7H15 M3554G3 53RV35 70 PR0V3 H0W 0UR M1ND5 C4N D0 4M4A1NG 7H1NG5! 1MPR3551V3 7H1NG5! 1N 7H3 B3G1NN1NG 17 WA5 H4RD BU7 N0W, 0N 7H15 L1N3, Y0UR M1ND 1S R34D1NG 17 4U70M471C4LL7 W17H0U7 3V3N 7HINK1NG 4B0U7 17.

If you didn't get this on the first read, it goes like this:

This message serves to prove how our minds can do amazing things! Impressive things! In the beginning, it was hard but now, on this line, your mind is reading it automatically without even thinking about it.

So, in the end, the conclusion remains that we don't believe what we see, we see what we want to believe.

And, so, we begin our journey into the world of evidence-based critical thinking.

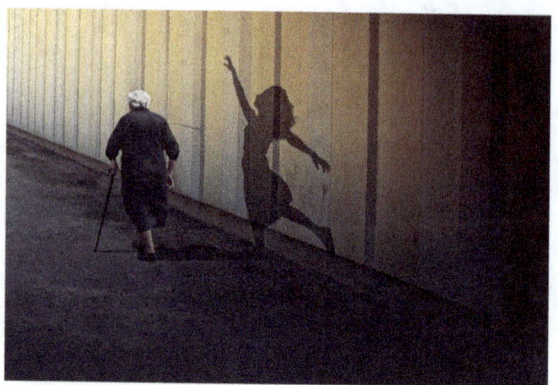

FIGURE 1.8 Dancing Shadow

Chapter 2

Understanding Evidence-Based Management

There was a great article published in the January 2006 issue of the *Harvard Business Review*, written by Jeffrey Pfeffer and Robert I. Sutton. They stated the following:

> At least since Plato's time, people have appreciated that true wisdom does not come from the sheer accumulation of knowledge, but from a healthy respect for and curiosity about the vast realms of knowledge still unconquered. Evidence-based management is conducted best not by know-it-alls but by managers who profoundly appreciate how much they do not know. These managers aren't frozen into inaction by ignorance; rather, they act on the best of their knowledge while questioning what they know.

Several years ago, my grandson, Oliver, was at my place helping me clear some trails on our property after a storm. I had the chainsaw and was cutting up the trees and limbs, and Oliver would help me load them onto the trailer. At one point, he just stopped and looked at me with those grandson eyes and said, "Poppy, I know everything." And I replied, "Really. About what?" and he said, "About everything." Now that's pretty cute when it comes from a six-year-old. But how about when it comes from your boss? Or you coworker? Or your spouse? Then it's no longer cute, it's just creepy! But we experience it all the time. Critical thinkers, those who move the world forward with creative and effective management results, know how much they do not know. The problem with being a know-it-all is that you are basically accepting the illusion that you have nothing more to learn. This means making decisions based on *a posteriori* knowledge, excluding the critically important process of considering new evidence.

While this technique can be applied in pretty much any environment or industry, healthcare presents us with its own unique challenges. For one, the level of criticality is often quite high; we are, after all, dealing with people's lives. Even from the perspective of non-clinical management, the decisions we make can impact the overall health of an entire community. I often ask this question when I am presenting at a conference: "What is the primary goal of a healthcare organization?" The answer I normally get is, "To provide quality care to our patients." While I am going to agree that this is certainly an important goal, I will opine that the primary goal is to be profitable. Let's face it, quality is expensive and unless you are the Federal Government, you can only operate at a deficit for so long before you simply go out of business. And if the organization closes, the community suffers, so financial viability has got to be our primary objective.

We also want to be able to increase access to care. I was recently engaged by a large health system that was experiencing problems with appointment gap times. This is the time between when the patient calls to make an appointment and when they are seen. For this practice, even for established patients, the gap time was more than six weeks. A non-evidence-based approach often adopted by the Centers for Medicare & Medicaid Services (CMS) would be to just throw money at the problem. Maybe hire a new provider.

But an evidence-based manager, a real critical thinker, would first convert this into a quantifiable problem. S/he would do some analysis, look at the data and the evidence, and conduct a cause-and-effect analysis, because if you don't know what is causing the problem, how can you expect to fix it? In this case, we found the no-show rate to be close to 20%. That meant that 1 out of 5 patients were simply not showing up for their appointment. When calculated out, this no-show rate accounted for nearly 4 weeks of the 6-week gap time. That means that, if we could figure out a way to fix this problem, we could reduce the gap time to 2 weeks. And that would solve more than just the gap problem, as we are about to see.

Four weeks of lost income for this practice amounted to several hundreds of thousands of dollars. Plus, there was a paradoxical issue that became apparent as we studied the problem. The extended lag time was responsible for the high no-show rate because as the lag time increases, so does the no-show rate. But the no-show rate resulted in an increase in lag time; or at least access, because there were hundreds of slots available for patients where no patient was available. In one case study, we found that appointments with a lead time of less than a week had a 4% no-show rate. Appointments with a 1- to 2-week lag time had an 8% no show rate. But once the lag time exceeded 3 weeks, the no-show rate doubled to just shy of 16% and at 6 weeks, it was close to 40%. Long lag times increased no-show rates and no-show rates increased lag time and reduced access. A real dilemma. So, what to do? They could just double up on appointments; that's an easy solution but would it work? Prior studies showed that this created more problems because, while it did fill some of the no-show slots, it also ended up overbooking way too many other slots, which increased wait time to the point that patients would walk out, resulting in the same problem as a no show: an empty appointment slot. To solve the problem, we looked at how others may have solved this problem and applied it to our data.

The airline industry has experienced this issue for some time and in only about 1 out of 20 instances is the plane overbooked. That's good, because overbooking a plane means that someone gets bumped and that is both expensive and bad PR. The airlines used a fairly complex model to calculate how many no-shows and last-minute cancellations occurred by location, time, and destination and came up with a very successful model. There was no reason we could not do the same and in fact, we did. I conducted an analysis of no-shows by provider and by time of day. In this case, I broke the day into four buckets: early morning (from 0800 to 1000), late morning (from 1000 to noon), early afternoon (from 1300 to 1500) and late afternoon (from 1500 to 1700). Using logistic regression, I was able to model the no-show problem and by applying basic statistics, created an appointment schedule that overbooked certain time slots for specific physicians on specific days. As it turned out, it worked. It reduced the lag time by 3 ½ weeks and in only 3% of appointment times was there an issue with double booking. Evidence. Data. Analytics. All these worked to the benefit of managing this issue and coming up with a positive, verifiable solution that could be validated moving forward.

Evidence-based management in a healthcare organization can also be employed to minimize regulatory and audit risk. I have spent the past six years working on an application that, using predictive modeling, can assess the likelihood that a billing/coding audit will occur, and if it does, which specific providers and/or procedures are the most likely targets. Called *risk-based auditing*, it involves the use of data and analytics to form its conclusions. This is what evidence-based management is all about. *Probe audits*, which are nothing more than a strategy of hoping to identify risk through some random process, is an example of anecdotal management. Hey, it worked in the past so maybe it will work in the future. NOT! This type of traditional thinking is the antithesis of critical thinking and can result in negative outcomes. Certainly not the career path of a successful manager.

About the Evidence

Several years ago, I attended a conference on problem solving. Let me get this out in the open now: I love problem solving. I have an entire library of books on complex problem solving and that is my bedtime reading. Story problems, logic problems, combinatoric and probability problems; if it's a problem, I'm your guy. In fact, if you were to ask any of my daughters what their dad does for a living, they would likely tell you that he solves people's problems. Now, I am not a 'soft tools' kind of guy. In fact, I teach a course on team building, but it isn't one of those soft and fuzzy team building courses, it is based on the use of heuristic modeling and the diversity prediction theorem. In my course, I teach organizations how to quantify the effectiveness of teams for problems solving and new program development. And it's all based on the evidence.

Well, the course on problem solving at this conference was a bit 'softer' than I am used to but, hey, I'm open to new ideas, so I attended. During the presentation, the instructor invited two people up to the podium and had them stand opposing each other, face-to-face. Then he pulled out a quarter and held it between them. He asked the man on the left what he saw, and then the woman on the right what she saw.

The man said, "George Washington."

And the woman said, "An eagle."

So, he saw the heads and she saw the tails. The instructor said that they were looking at the same problem from different perspectives. The solution he offered was to look at the coin, if you will, from the same side.

I didn't think much of the session but one day, a few months later, I was having a disagreement with my wife about something, and I had this great idea. I pulled out a quarter from my pocket and held it up to her.

I said, "Honey, what do you see?"

And she said, "An idiot holding a quarter."

The moral of the story? Not every tool works every time, so it is important to make sure that you have a toolbox with the requisite tools necessary to work through your problems. This is Ashby's Law of Requisite Variety, and stand by, because I am going to discuss that in detail later.

In considering the evidence, we need to face the issue of the Law of Diminishing Returns. In general, this measures the point at which the cost in energy or money invested begins to exceed the benefits expected or realized. According to businessdictionary.com, the Law of Diminishing Returns is, "A concept in economics that if one factor of production (number of workers, for example) is increased while other factors (machines and workspace, for example) are held constant, the output per unit of the variable factor will eventually diminish."

From our perspective, it means that there is a point at which the cost of information begins to exceed the benefit of its purpose. For example, it may cost a provider 15% of their revenue to collect 97% of what they are due from third party payers. But it may cost another 25% to collect the remaining 3%, which diminishes the value of the remaining amount. In the area of analytics, information tends to scale exponentially. For example, to double the amount of good information I need, I may have to square the cost. It becomes incumbent upon the evidence-based manager to balance evidence against cost to ensure the most positive result with the most efficient and cost-effective process.

We also need to balance the value of information. We all know that there is a cost for valuable information. It may be in the form of time, effort, resources, dollars, or all the above. But we should also be aware that there is a greater cost for bad information. Let's say that I have a final in the morning and it is all true or false questions. Rather than study that night, I went out and partied, so I don't have a clue as to the answer. Probabilistically speaking, if I close my eyes and guess, my score will float around 50%. That's chance. Now let's say that I study all night, but it's with someone that doesn't like me, so they feed me the incorrect information. Now, it is much more likely that my score will be below 50% or chance, because I am going into the exam with bad information.

Chapter 3

Paper or Plastic?

It may have been the most mind-boggling, flabbergasting moment in our married life for my wife when I told her that I was going to teach a course on decision making. She was beside herself, because I have not proven to be the best decision maker around the house. I mean, when it comes to my work, I do an excellent job. In fact, people pay me for my problem-solving skills. My work requires me to come out on top with effective decisions derived from complex information. But it's the simple things that seem to knock me through a loop. Given the requisite data for a post-audit extrapolation assessment, I can usually come up with a successful challenge within a few hours of analysis. But when I get to the check-out at the local grocery store and they ask me if I want paper or plastic, I fall into a fetal ball and begin to mumble. I don't know how to choose because I have never taken the time to assess the differences between the two. There are lots of considerations, like environmental (paper degrades, plastic does not), value (paper is more expensive), reuse (plastic will last longer), utility (which will hold and transport groceries better), & etc. It is my opinion that, in general, people overestimate both the complexity of decision making as well as their own abilities at making good decisions.

What is a decision, anyway? Well, as stated earlier, it is a conclusion we draw upon to take some action. I think one of the greatest fallacies about decision-making is that there are some people who are just naturally great decision-makers. People who tend to make good decisions on a regular basis have a strong background of experiential *learning* often paired with formal *training* in decision modeling. Not through natural ability. And contrary to widespread belief, decisions are rarely made on the spot but are made based on accumulated information collected over some time. For example, a manager who might make what appears to be an on the spot decision about a particular issue or problem has likely been exposed to that issue or problem over time and has had the opportunity to review data and evidence as it pertains to that issue or problem.

Professor Barbara Sahakian and Jamie Nicole LaBuzetta, in a study they reported in their book *Bad Moves: How Decision Making Goes Wrong, and the Ethics of Smart Drugs*, estimated that the average adult makes around 35,000 *remotely conscious decisions* each day. A study published in the journal *Environment and Behavior* in January 2007 by Brian Wansink and Jeffery Sobal, of Cornell University, showed that we make over 225 decisions each day on food alone. And I love that this sort of decision making is called *remotely conscious*. What does that even mean? I think this is important to understand because we often see decision making as a cognitive process but that is not always the case. In making decisions, we are rarely faced with only one viable option. In fact, good decision-making is the ability to cognitively select between a series of alternatives. Obviously, our goal is to pick the best alternative. We want our decisions to be defensible as well. In my work, the necessity to defend my decisions is critical. In fact, I often must defend those decisions in front of a judge or jury.

Just think about what's involved in making a decision to cross a busy street. First, you assess your physical capabilities. Can you even make it across the street without falling or running out of breath? To assess this, you must calculate the distance to cross the road. Let's say it's a divided four-lane road. Each lane is about 12 feet wide and the median is also about 12 feet wide. So, to get from one side to the other is about 60 feet and just to make it to the median is about 24 feet. Next, you must estimate how quickly you can move. One study estimates that a healthy adult will walk across a street at a crosswalk at the rate of about 4 ½ ft/s. That means it would take you about five seconds to make it to the median and about 14 seconds to get all the way across the street.

Next, you must determine whether there's any traffic. And if there is, you must estimate the velocity. For example, are there cars moving toward you or away from you? Are they accelerating, decelerating, or remaining at the constant speed? Do you have a backup plan in case something goes wrong? For example, if you trip and fall or if a car comes out of another street that you didn't see, or a vehicle begins to accelerate that wasn't accelerating when you stepped into the street? Suffice it to say that most of these decisions are remotely conscious. They are almost automatic. If you took the time to do all this math with your calculator, by the time you're ready to step into the street, all the conditions would've changed, because crossing a street invokes a dynamic state: all the parameters are changing all the time.

How about making a decision to go to work in the morning? Maybe you have an alarm clock. The decision about what time to set it for originated at least the night before, so this decision spans a greater amount of time. The alarm goes off, and you have a decision to make. Do you turn it off and get up? Do you turn it off and go back to sleep? Maybe you hit the snooze button. What data and information goes into making this first quite simple decision? Well, is it a workday? Can you afford to take a day off? If you hit the snooze button, will that make you late? Or maybe you'll get a few more minutes of sleep, but you won't be able to get a cup of coffee or make breakfast. What about breakfast? What information do we need to make that decision? Are you hungry? Do you have food to make breakfast? Do you have time to prepare breakfast? And even the type of breakfast that you are going to eat is dependent upon time. Do you have time to take a shower? Do you need one? If each of these decision points were totally cognitive—meaning you calculated each one consciously—you would never get anything done. In fact, you would suffer from what I call "paralysis of analysis." I will explain that in greater detail later but suffice it to say that, at some point, we are subject to decision fatigue. We can burn out from an overwhelming decision-making process.

The University of Massachusetts Dartmouth has put together a seven-step decision-making process. It goes like this:

A Seven Step Decision-Making Process

Step 1: Identify the decision

Step 2: Gather relevant information

Step 3: Identify alternatives

Step 4: Weigh the evidence

Step 5: Choose among alternatives

Step 6: Take action

Step 7: Review your decision

Identify the decision and gather relevant information

The first question that we need to ask ourselves is, do we even need to make a decision here? And, if so, what is the purpose and the nature of the decision that we must make? That is Step 1. Then we have Step 2, which goes to the core of what I am talking about in this book. We need to collect information that is relevant to our decision. This step is often harder than it seems. I am an older guy now, and I can tell you that when I was a younger guy, my biggest problem was getting access to enough information. Today, the problem is that there is too much information and sorting through it to separate useful from worthless is difficult. In fact, we often must deal with *asymmetry of information.*

In contract theory, asymmetry of information is a situation where one person or party has more or better information that another person or party. We find this occurs quite often when we go to the vendor hall at some of our larger conferences. You may have a dozen vendors there that are selling electronic health records (EHR) applications or practice management systems. Each of those vendors is going to have data and other information that prove they are the best. But logically, we know that not everyone could be the best. If we are lazy, this becomes a problem. But if we are serious about the decisions we are going to make, like spending a fortune on an EHR, then we must be committed to doing research beyond just what the vendor is willing to give us. Remember, this is what they do for a living, so asymmetry results because they likely will have more information than you do. But with a little effort, you can solve that problem.

Identify alternatives

In Step 3, we are going to look at alternatives for our decisions. For example, in the appointment lead time problem covered earlier, there were several alternatives for solving the problem. We could address the no-show issue, or we could hire another provider. We might even consider increasing the physical space or converting nontreatment rooms into treatment rooms. In any case, management decision is going to entail assessing alternatives.

Weigh the evidence

Step 4 is obviously my favorite, which is weighing the evidence. Now remember, much of how we measure the success and outcomes of our decisions will be based on the quality of the data and evidence that we consider. I will discuss this in much greater detail later.

In general, I like to come in with a null hypothesis. In statistics, null hypotheses usually state that sample observations or data result purely from chance. In a criminal trial, the null hypothesis is that the person is not guilty. It is rare to have enough evidence to clearly state that a person is innocent, only a lack of evidence to say that the person is guilty. The same is true in our decisions. We rarely have enough information to say that this is the correct decision, but rather, to say that it's the least incorrect decision based on the available evidence. So, in our example of appointment lag time, the null hypothesis would be that it is just a result of chance occurrence. The alternate hypothesis might be that it is a result of a high no-show rate. The purpose of examining the evidence is to determine whether we reject that null hypothesis. We either *have* enough evidence to say that it's not true, or we *don't have* enough evidence to say that it is not true. But rarely do we have enough evidence to say that it is in fact 100% true.

Choose among alternatives, take action, and review your decision

Once we have weighed the evidence, we can go to Step 5 and look at the different alternatives and determine which one we want to take. For example, let's say that we have a problem with excessive wait time before patient sees the doctor. This might be due to a number of reasons. It could be that the doctor comes in late. Or it could be that patients are sicker than average. It might also be that patients come in for their appointment too early and therefore add waiting time that is outside the scope of their appointment time. It could be that it's due to patient age and their inability to show up on time, or due to an unusual mix of new patients versus established patients. In some cases, it may be that the new patient intake process is longer than it should be. What we are setting out here are several different hypotheses, with the null hypothesis being that excessive waiting time just occurs as a matter of chance. We examine the evidence, and our goal. Rather than finding the correct alternative, we may be able to eliminate the incorrect alternatives as a more efficient way to solve our problem.

To do this, we would conduct a study. First, we might take some sample of patients each day for thirty days to calculate the actual waiting time. And if we do this correctly, we would be able to stratify by time of day, day of week, age of patient, status as new or established patient and even by provider. By doing this, we would be able to eliminate those alternatives not supported by the evidence. What we are left with is the probable cause. So, we choose amongst our alternatives and, Step 6, act to correct the problem. Later in this book, I will get into the details of problem solving, which will address *how* we take action and validate our results. Finally, Step 7, we want to review our decision. This doesn't mean that we all get together and either have a high five or a thumbs down party. This step is a review of the evidence to either validate or invalidate the outcomes of our decision. And again, I will get into this in much greater detail in the section on problem-solving.

How Are Decisions Really Made?

These seven steps represent an accepted formal decision-making process. But how are decisions really made? Particularly when we are dealing with the enterprise or organizational level? For sure, many of us make decisions based on intuition. It feels right so it must be right. And we all have stories about how that model failed us miserably. We make decisions based on emotion. My dad always told me not to make a decision when I was hungry, angry, lonely, or tired. He felt doing so would introduce individual decision biases that would almost guarantee making the wrong decision.

We also make decisions based on our own personal survival. I have been in more than a few situations where people made decisions based on the impact on their jobs of a new program or technology. In some situations, employees would attempt to sabotage a management decision to save their own skin. And while I understand why someone might do this, it does not lend itself toward positive outcomes.

We also make decisions based on politics, particularly in larger organizations. Some decisions are more politically expedient than others and in some cases our jobs may depend on which end of the political spectrum we support.

We also make decisions based on anecdote, which we have already discussed. And, on the positive side, we will base our decisions on prior experience. While this is not all bad, an experience may not correlate as much as we might imagine to our current situation. Although the problems may look the same, there may be different root causes, and cause-and-effect is a critical part of decision-making. Most of our decisions contain parts of the above. Instead of basing our decisions on these considerations, we want our decision-making to be based on *unbounded rationality*. Unbounded rationality is decision-making that favors logic, analysis, evidence, and objectivity over the subjectivity, intuition, and anecdote of *bounded rationality*.

Herbert Simon is Chaired Professor in psychology and computer science at Carnegie Mellon University, an economist and political scientist whose research focused mostly on the science of decision-making. He received the Nobel Prize in Economics in 1978, the Turing award in 1975, and was a leader and pioneer in the areas of decision-making, problem-solving, artificial intelligence, and complex systems. He was a guru amongst economists. In 1956, he published an article on unbounded rationality and concluded that most people make decisions with limited knowledge of all the options available. In 1947, he published the first edition of his book called *Administrative Behavior: A Study of Decision-Making Processes in Administrative Organizations*. I recommend that anyone who is interested in the topic of decision-making reads the fourth edition of this book, which was published in 1997. His thesis is that, "Decision-making is at the heart of administration and that the vocabulary of administrative theory must be derived from logic and psychology of human choice."

This idea of bounded rationality encroaches on every aspect of our lives. A good example of this occurs in the voting booth. In our most recent election in Florida, not only did we have an election for governor, senator, and several congressional positions, but there were also thirteen state amendments on the ballot. For example, Amendment 6 added a Marcy's law to the Florida Constitution, increasing judicial retirement age to 75, and prohibiting judges from deferring to administrative agencies in interpreting the law. Amendment 10 prohibited counties from abolishing certain local offices, changing start dates of legislative sessions, and added an executive office of the executive department to the constitution. And while most people had enough information to make an educated decision about their vote for governor, or senator, or maybe even Congress, very few had the information necessary to make an educated decision regarding these and the dozens of other amendments that appeared on local ballots. But they voted for them anyway. In some studies, we find that just the way an amendment is named has a significant impact on a person's decision. The sad part is that we are making decisions, voting on things that may have a significant impact in our lives, with only a limited knowledge of all the options available.

Randall Bartlett, Professor of Economics at Smith College, coined *the blind-date principle*, which is a corollary to bounded rationality.

In his book *Economic Foundations of Political Power*, Professor Bartlett gives this example:

> My cousin is coming to town and would like a date for the weekend. I supply you with information that he has a spectacular personality, an exceptional sense of humor, and gorgeous, deep blue eyes. I neglect to mention that he has three of them, travels on a motorized pogo stick, and has several highly communicable diseases. By intentionally biasing the stock of information I can lead you to make a choice you might not have made in the absence of my persuasion. I have changed your behavior. I have affected your lifetime utility (in this case presumably negatively).

We need to recognize that any information we don't generate ourselves comes from someone else, such as vendors, the government, research organizations, etc. We also need to recognize that purveyors of information usually have an incentive to use the information under their control to try to influence our decisions. The most effective solution to this problem is to, at the very least, recognize that this condition exists. In that way, even the information we receive is quite asymmetrical, we can, as the U.S. Marines say, "Improvise, adapt, overcome."

Strategies versus tactics

Before we discuss the levels of decision making, I wanted to touch on two decision concepts: strategies and tactics. These two terms are often confused, but there is a world of difference between the two. *Strategy* describes the long-term objective or global plan for an organization or individual. *Tactics* are the step-by-step actions taken to meet a short-term goal or objective that can be a part of a given strategy. Let's look at the game of chess as an example. Statisticians have calculated that, in a standard game of chess that involves 40 paired moves, there are 10 to the 120th power of move combinations. That means that, in a game with 64 squares and 32 pieces, there are more moves than there are protons in the known universe. The strategy, or long-term objective, is to win the game. The tactics describe each move. In a strategy, you may have your mind set on a particular opening or middle game, but tactically, each move must accomplish a more immediate goal. Strategically, I was taught that there are three priorities in playing chess:

1. **Forcing moves first:** These moves leave the opponent with as little choice as possible.
2. **Direct threats:** These are moves that threaten and are generally not as forcing as checks and captures.
3. **Positional moves:** These are moves that improve your position, strengthen a weak point, restrict enemy pieces, and in general, help your strategic plan.

Tactics, however, take on a completely different view. For example, before making any given move, I would want to consider the following:

1. Is anything in danger?
2. Who controls the square where I want to move?
3. What was the response to my last move?
4. Does my move help me or my opponent?
5. Does my move solve the problem(s) created by my opponent's last move?
6. And finally, what is my plan for the next move?

My first chess instructor told me that chess moves are like musical notes. How they fit together will decide whether you create a melody or just a bunch of noise. I would opine that the tactics we employ in decision making create the same situation. Tactics, when properly strung together, are critical to supporting our longer-term strategic objectives. It is also important to note that, while strategic decisions are normally quite stable, tactical decisions can change based on the dynamic nature of a given system or state. In essence, shift happens! Expect the unexpected and you will be disappointed less often than not.

The Three Levels of Decision Making

There are three levels of decision making;

1. **Individual** (includes day-to-day decisions involving family, career, etc.)
2. **Group** (occurs within teams and can be both personal and professional)
3. **Corporate** (involves organizations with both political and social influence)

For the purposes of this book, I am going to focus mostly on the individual decision-making level. I will discuss how to build effective decision-making teams and their associated biases later in the book.

Let's start by discussing individual decision biases. If you were to look cognitive biases up in, say, Wikipedia, you would find more than one hundred under the heading "Decision-making, belief, and behavioral biases." It's more than I can manage. So, I am going to look at the five I believe are the most significant for individual decision making.

The first is the *overconfidence effect*, supported by the *Dunning-Kruger effect*. The overconfidence effect, or bias, is almost self-explanatory. It means that we are more confident in our abilities or decisions than is supported by objective assessment. Overconfidence not only impacts our management and business decisions but can also be dangerous, as it causes us to believe we can do something that we can't, like climb a mountain or outrun a moose! The Dunning-Kruger effect, also a cognitive bias, leads us to imagine our abilities are greater than they are. In fact, there is an interesting paradox regarding the Dunning-Kruger effect where our illusion of competence actually inhibits our ability to see our incompetence, further aggravating the consequences of our actions.

Inversely, the Dunning-Kruger effect also describes that highly competent people will underestimate their abilities. William Shakespeare may have put it best in *As You Like It* when he had Touchstone say, "The fool doth think he is wise, but the wise man knows himself to be a fool."

Bertrand Russell, a 20th century philosopher and mathematician once said, "One of the painful things about our time is that those who feel certainty are stupid, and those with any imagination and understanding are filled with doubt and indecision." It would serve us well to heed to these writings.

The *sunk cost bias* (or fallacy) may well be one of the most consequential of the individual cognitive biases. From my experience, this single bias is the greatest impediment to growth and positive fulfillment of strategic objectives. A sunk cost, by definition, is a cost that has already been incurred and is, so to speak, permanently lost or unrecoverable. Sometimes, this is referred to as a *sunk-cost trap*, which, according to Investopedia.com, ". . . refers to a tendency for people to irrationally follow through on an activity that is not meeting their expectations. This is because of the time and/or money they have already invested."

Perhaps the most famous example of this is the failed Mt. Everest expeditions of 1996, chronicled in detail in the book *Into Thin Air* by Jon Krakauer. I am going to avoid a detailed reliving of the event, but I do think that a summary is in order here. The year 1996, saw the third highest number of deaths recorded in a single day in the history of Mt. Everest climbs. In all, eight climbers died, and many others stranded and injured because of poor decision making on the part of both participants and expedition leaders. In general, there was an agreement amongst the climbers that they would turn around and head back down the mountain at a certain time whether or not they had reached the summit. But when that time came, several climbers decided to continue on, even though it put their lives and the lives of their guides in jeopardy. Why?

Well, many believe it was due to the sunk cost bias. These climbers invested tens of thousands of dollars in permit and guide fees. They had to commit three to six months of their lives to even think about climbing Mt. Everest. They invested time and effort over several months just to properly acclimate to the altitude and rigor of the climb. And, after all that, after sinking all that cost into an event with a single goal in mind, which was to reach the summit, turning around when the summit was in view was simply not an option. The result was that people were willing to risk their lives rather than suffer the irrecoverable loss of the investments they made into the trip.

I see this problem quite frequently when working with healthcare providers. For example, I worked with a larger enterprise organization that had a terrible EHR system. They struggled to produce even the most basic data needed to create operational analyses and reports. But they were not interested in looking into newer and more data-centric systems because they had already "sunk" so much time, money, and training into this system. They were willing to sacrifice their ability to improve operational efficiency, increase access to care, and reduce compliance risk because of an irrecoverable cost. What a shame!

The habit of assessing a situation by what comes most easily to mind is the *availability bias* (or *availability heuristic*). The tendency to make decisions or form opinions based on the information that is readily available is, in *my* opinion, evidence of profound cognitive laziness. For example, someone may have spent a few weeks in Florida when the weather was unseasonably hot and humid (if that is even a real thing!), and as result, decide not to return to Florida again, believing that every period in the future would be just like that period in the past. I have heard it said that we tend to judge any group of people by its least favorable members and forming judgments of groups this way is an example of the availability bias. The Joint Commission published a *Quick Safety* article (Issue 28, October 2016) that includes, amongst others, mention of availability bias. The article defines it as, "Judging likelihood of a diagnosis based on the ease with which examples can be retrieved (more familiar, common, recent, memorable) (e.g., diagnosing a patient based on frequently seen conditions such as the flu, or not considering less common diagnoses)."

From a manager's perspective, I have seen decisions made about technology based solely on readily available information (maybe from a vendor) or the experiences of just a handful of folks. Clinically, availability bias is responsible for many instances of misdiagnoses, as discussed in the above referenced article and, administratively, is responsible for many poor decisions regarding technology as well as staff employment. The solution to this bias is to spend more time and energy researching alternative data sources rather than complacently taking only data that is readily available or anecdotal.

A cousin of availability bias is *confirmation bias*. Confirmation bias is the tendency to interpret new evidence (or look for existing evidence and information) that confirms our pre-existing theories, theses, or beliefs. For example, I know someone who won't even consider quitting smoking because his grandfather lived to be ninety-seven and smoked his entire adult life. Forget about the thousands of studies that show just how bad smoking is for us. The same goes for, say, drinking coffee. There are a hundred studies that say coffee is good for you and a hundred that say it's bad. We tend to focus on those studies that support our preferences so, if I like to drink coffee, I focus on those that say it is good for me. Period.

Here's an example from my own personal life. My wife believes that I regularly (or always) leave the toilet seat up. I, on the other hand, believe that it is a rarity, an anomaly, if you will. Under the influence of confirmation bias, she does not notice when the seat is down, only when the seat is up. So, if I leave the seat up, say, once a week, that confirms for her that I leave the seat up "all the time." In defense of my position, I put a clipboard next to the toilet, and every time she used the bathroom, she would place a check in one box if the seat was up and in the other box if it was down. Truth be told, it was more than once a week but certainly much less than "all the time."

I have encountered this cognitive bias numerous times when working with healthcare organizations. In one engagement, leadership wanted to install an electronic prescription software system. Their goal was to improve the prescribing process, reduce prescribing errors, and take advantage of additional reimbursement from Medicare. The downside was that there was quite a bit of evidence within the community that these types of applications resulted in, at the very least, an initial reduction in productivity. The problem was convincing the physician leadership that the small potential increase in revenue (which, by the way, they would never see) was worth the decrease in productivity and the hassle of learning yet another new technology.

In the end, it was my opinion that the organization was not ready to implement an e-prescribe system. They disagreed and terminated my engagement. Then, they brought on another consultant who agreed with them that it was a promising idea and that they were, in fact, ready. They went ahead with implementation. It was an abject failure, resulting in lost productivity, revenue, and physician confidence in leadership. Hopefully, you can see how confirmation bias played into their decision. Unbeknownst to me, they had already decided that they were going to move forward with this plan before they engaged me, and all they were looking for was someone to confirm their beliefs and communicate those effectively to the medical staff. When I wouldn't do it, they found someone who would.

Michael Shermer, publisher of the magazine *Skeptic*, in a piece published in the Huffington Post, wrote "Being deeply knowledgeable on one subject narrows one's focus and increases confidence, but it also blurs dissenting views until they are no longer visible, thereby transforming data collection into bias confirmation and morphing self-deception into self-assurance." 'nough said!

Finally, there is framing *bias*. This describes a bias that develops from how information is framed, or, in other words, how it is presented to us. I believe that we have all seen this, particularly from vendors. They tend to have highly polished graphic presentations with evidence, data, and information that supports their positions. They present it in such a way as to convince us that their solution is the correct solution, and that it will result in higher productivity, lower cost, and less risk, when in fact the opposite may be true. Framing bias is great if you are selling something but not so great if you are buying. I have, in the past, been up against other consultants in responding to a request for proposal (RFP) and, even though my fee may have been lower and my services more superior, they got the gig because their presentation was prettier. The problem is that relying on external cues like this can easily skew the decision-making logic that we so desperately seek.

As an example, imagine being faced with the need to move more aggressively into risk-based auditing, so you start a search for applications and systems that can help you with this strategic objective. In the context of framing bias, the presenter might compare the current state with a state that was riskier, even if this is not the best comparison. For example, they might say something like, "CMS reports that audit recovery increased three-fold over the past five years." Rather than saying, "Audit recovery increased by 12.5% over the past year." The former, while *not untrue*, gives the (false) impression of a significantly higher risk of recovery than the change over the past year. Presenting the comparison over the past year would indicate a significant slow-down in recovery, resulting in reduced risk and result in a reduced sense of urgency on the part of the client. While both statistics are true, how someone frames risk can have a huge impact on the decision-making process.

Decision Theory

In both simple and complex systems, we see decision theory centering around two primary concepts: *uncertainty* and *risk*. Uncertainly is a probabilistic problem in which the possible outcome (or outcomes) are measured in distributions. Like reporting the weather, we are trying to determine the probability an event is likely to occur. In weather forecasting, for example, what does a 40% chance of rain mean? It could mean that they are 100% confident it will rain in 40% of the coverage area. Or it could mean that they are 40% confident it will rain at least somewhere within the coverage area. Or it could mean that they are 80% confident that it will rain in 50% of the coverage area. The prediction is based on a combination of data points meant to express the underlying uncertainty and risk.

Risk assesses the likelihood that an outcome will result in some loss to the system. For example, if you are thinking of hiring a PA or NP, risk could be measured by the probability that patients won't accept him or her or that some of the payers may not reimburse for some of his or her services. Risk must be quantified if we are to develop expected value calculations or even model ROI. The fact is, there is risk in every decision and every action, no matter how small. In some cases, the risk can be high but the cost low, while in other situations, the risk can be low, but the cost can be astronomical. This ability to absorb the cost of failure or a negative outcome is "utility," and it is an often-ignored component of decision making. Utility describes how able the system is to absorb the risk. For example, a twenty-five-physician practice may not blink at the potential loss of hiring a PA who doesn't work out, while a three-physician practice might reel from the potential scheduling and financial consequences.

Without considering uncertainty, we end up with a deterministic model, producing the same output for a given input without consideration for risk or uncertainty. Let's look at how this might impact a real-world example. If I were to produce a fair coin, we could be confident that, when flipped, that coin would land heads up half the time and tails up half the time. In this case, we know that the probability of a heads or a tail is 50%, so the uncertainty is locked in for our purposes. Now let's say that you and I turn this into a betting game, and for each flip, you pay me a quarter if it's heads or I pay you a quarter if it's tails. How likely would you be to play this game with me? First, we address risk: you have a 50% chance of losing a quarter with each flip. If you were to end up losing ten, your "risk" would be a loss of $2.50. Finally, we must deal with utility, which is your ability to manage, or to survive the impact of that risk. I would guess that both you and I could survive a $2.50 expenditure.

Let's play the same game again, but this time, we bet $10,000 each flip, so if you were to experience a net loss of ten flips in this game, the risk is losing $250,000. Who wants to play now? Even if you said you wanted to, I wouldn't, because, from the utility perspective, I simply cannot afford to lose a quarter of a million dollars, especially flipping coins! Notice that the uncertainty has not changed; we still have a 50/50 probability of heads or tails. The risk has not change; each of us still runs the risk of losing some amount of money with some known probability. What has changed is the utility: our ability to absorb the loss due to the risk.

The Four Levels of Uncertainty

Let's draw our attention back to the issue of uncertainty. Based on a great article entitled "Strategy Under Uncertainty" by Hugh Courtney, Jane Kirkland, and Patrick Viguerie, there are four definable levels of uncertainty:

- Level 1 represents a clear and singular future.
- Level 2 represents alternative future scenarios.
- Level 3 represents a wide range of futures, some of which can be ambiguous.
- Level 4 represents true ambiguity or an uncertainty that may not be discoverable.

Let's look at each of these in greater detail:

Level 1 – A Clear Future

Level 1 events are found in simple, non-complex (linear) systems. A limited set of key variables produces few uncertainty distributions. It is a single, linear look into the future. Predictions are easy to make. We are confident in both the consequences of a decision and the likelihood of occurrence. From a mathematical perspective, data for Level 1 events usually work with point estimates, a single forecast, such as a trend analysis, and confidence intervals. A potential Level 1 event in a medical practice is hiring a new provider. It is straightforward to analyze patient flow, wait time, room turnaround time, and lag times to appointments. In this case, we might see that average wait time exceeds forty-five minutes and it takes more than three weeks for a new patient to see a provider. In this case, while there may be other reasons for these metrics, we could, easily measure the uncertainty, risk, and utility.

The key here is predictability. For example, it is likely that the practice has brought on a new provider in the past and can use the data from that event to predict the outcome for this event. That may include looking at visit ramp-up times, break-even dates, etc.

Level 2 – Alternative Futures

In Level 2 scenarios, we may have a few different views of the future. While we don't really know for certain which of those views will eventually happen, we can (as you will see shortly) assign some probability to each. We will build an expected value calculation, of sorts, to assess likelihood of occurrence as well as magnitude of risk. There are Level 2 events in both simple and complex systems. We have seen this scenario play out multiple times over the past twenty years or so regarding Medicare fees. Often, the final fee schedule is held political hostage to some other agenda, and, in the past, the final rule wasn't published until after the first of the year, the threshold for when it should have taken effect. This leaves the practice to guess as to what the fee schedule will look like. When Medicare makes up a sizable portion of your revenues, say more than 25%, uncertainty can be a killer. In general, Level 2 scenarios play out when there are multiple actors and we don't have enough information on any of the actors to be able to predict their behavior. In this case, each actor has their own uncertainty curve and the trick is to be able to predict the likelihood that each scenario plays out and to have a plan for each one.

A good example of this would be implementation of an EHR. A few years ago, we conducted a study to find out perception vs. reality of integrating an EHR into a healthcare organization. We asked those who had not yet purchased an EHR how long they thought full integration would take and the approximate average guess was six months. Then, we asked those who had fully integrated how long it took them. The approximate average was two years. The focus of the gap appeared to be the uncertainties for each of the actors involved in the integration process. There was the vendor, who had their agenda and time objectives. There were the providers, who had their own issues regarding integration and ways to mitigate productivity loss. We also had to deal with the training and staff availability, and on and on and on. For each vector, we needed to estimate the time-to-completion, the costs involved, contingency plans (I will discuss this in detail later), failure nodes, and even try to "imagine" things that could go wrong.

Level 3 – Alternate Futures

At Level 3, we will be met with a range of possible futures occurring in complex systems, since the degree of uncertainty is often defined as a group of disparate and often non-communicative players. While the mechanics are not much different than what we face at Level 2, the predicates are. Here, unlike in Level 2 uncertainty, there are no natural scenarios. This means that, even though we can often think through different futures, it is difficult to determine which to develop more completely based on some realistic expectation of the outcomes. When modeling the uncertainty, probability curves may resemble one another, exacerbating the problem. At Level 2, we can imagine some discrete outcomes, while at Level 3 we are just trying to ensure movement so we can modify the plan as we move through the state.

If there is a benefit to Level 3 uncertainties, it is that we usually have some past event to study. For example, for those of us steeped in healthcare, an example of an event at this level was the changeover from ICD-9 to ICD-10. Not because we can predict the entire range of futures, but because those of us that have been around long enough have seen these transitions occur in the past so even though, in this case, that may not be the best predictor, it is a predictor, nonetheless. Moving forward, we may be a bit hamstrung, craving more evidence that may be available and end up inserting our intuition where we would normally insert probability models.

Another example that is fresh on all our minds was the proposed changes for 2019 to the E&M codes for physician services. CMS was proposing to go from a five-level model to a two-level model that, in the end, proved to be a bit too radical and unsustainable for immediate implementation. Instead, they postponed the change until 2021, but it's anyone's guess what it will really look like then. In the meantime, it is prudent to begin to, at the very least, create a set of futures for how a change such as that will impact your practice. There are those of us (likely now grandparents) who remember the changeover in 1992, from the old model (i.e. 99002) to the new model (i.e. 99213) for coding E&M codes. It moved from an intuitive system to one that was defined by specific quantifiable standards, which changed, by the way, over the subsequent few years. Those of use that were around for that may have a better idea of what to expect in the future, predicting the probabilities surrounding those uncertainties and being able to imagine a broader range of futures.

Level 4 – True Ambiguity

Level 4 uncertainty states are found in highly complex systems. Not only is it difficult to imagine a set of futures, since there is little to nothing in the past to assist with forecasting, it is about impossible to model the probabilities and even risk. In some circles, a Level 4 event is a "black swan," or an event that is rare, unpredictable, and followed by significant impact or consequences. Black swan events can be either negative or positive but are pretty much always a surprise.

One example might be the Deepwater Horizon oil spill that began in April of 2010, in the Gulf of Mexico. The government estimated that some 4.9 million barrels (210 million gallons) leaked into the gulf, resulting in extensive damage to marine and wildlife habitat. If imagining that future isn't hard enough, imagine trying to predict, in advance, the impact on the fishing and tourism industry. The fact is, no one had ever imagined a spill of this magnitude, so it took everyone by surprise. That means that there wasn't any specific strategy to manage a situation like that and, as a result, it was months before any corrective action proved beneficial. Over 2,000 tons of oil and oily material was removed from Louisiana beaches some three years later, in 2013. In the end, the courts ordered BP to pay $18.7 billion in fines, the largest corporate settlement at that time. Who would have predicted that?

Another example is the 9.1 magnitude earthquake that struck outside of Tokyo in March of 2011. Not only was the quake itself damaging, but it created a tsunami with 30-foot waves that damaged several nuclear reactors along the shoreline. It was, in fact, the largest earthquake ever to hit Japan and the next largest in recent history was an 8.6 that hit in 1707. Planning for a 9.1 and the possibility of a large magnitude tsunami was pretty much out of reach for most planners.

Even if someone had the forethought to predict this, imagining the futures it would create would be a near impossibility. First, predicting the tsunami. Then predicting the location of the tsunami and the impact it would have on the nuclear reactors. Moving forward, imagining the wider impact of having radioactive material transported across the Pacific Ocean past Hawaii and to Washington and California. I remember being in Hawaii a year or so after that and finding items on the beach that were clearly debris from that event.

On the positive side, the largest lottery jackpot ever was the $1.6 billion Powerball back in 2018. Taking the instant gratification option, that would pay out $905 million in one lump sum. I don't care who you are, no matter how hard you tried, you could never really imagine your set of futures from an event like that. Unless of course, you were already a billionaire!

In almost every Level 4 event that I have studied, decision capabilities were modeled after the fact. It's like writing a book about the ten things that haven't yet been discovered! It sounds preposterous, yet every decade or so, we are surprised by some massive black swan event. And while we can't prepare necessarily for the specific event, we can, using tools that I will discuss later, be prepared no matter what confronts us.

I think that one of the things that really distinguishes a Level 4 approach is that we go from a reliance on quantitative data to qualitative information. The best we can do is to maybe study how other industries have dealt with black swan events, even if the actual event does not represent what we are facing. For example, we can look at ACA as a Level 4 event. In 2010, Nancy Pelosi, the house minority leader at the time, said: "But we have to pass the bill so that you can find out what is in it, away from the fog of the controversy." She was saying that our ability to imagine what would be some realistic view of the future was hamstrung because, without passage, we had no clue what was in the bill and, hence, no clue of what to expect! Note that this is not a political statement but a management statement. Imagine trying to manage a large organization or department when told that you wouldn't know what was in your budget until after it had been approved! But, hey, I imagine that has, in fact, happened to some of you.

Asymmetry of Information

When considering the information that goes into making a decision, it is critical that we are able to identify the point of origination for the data and the evidence we are considering. As mentioned earlier, within the decision-making world, we must deal with asymmetry of information, to round out more fully our need to understand concepts of uncertainty and risk. In some circles, it is called *rational ignorance*, although asymmetry of information may be both an intentional and an unintentional consequence of evidence-based management. *Asymmetry of information* means that the information that we have, whether in the form of data or evidence or other materials, often comes from a source that has an incentive to use the information under their control to try to influence our decisions. In rational ignorance, this asymmetry occurs because we have determined that the cost of obtaining the information is greater than the benefit of what we might learn. Therefore, it becomes irrational to waste time and money and resources to gain that information.

This is most often the case when we visit vendors at one of our healthcare conferences. For example, there may be five or six vendors all selling EHR systems. Each vendor will present the information that identifies their product as the best, but we all know that not every one of them can be the best, especially in all areas. What they are doing is bending the data to reflect those areas around their product offering that may excel in one or more features. Sometimes this occurs because of withholding negative information, hence the use of the word 'asymmetry.' We might also see this occur quite commonly in elections, where candidates will each provide information that proves they are the best choice for the voter. Rational ignorance is when we choose not to learn about all the items on the ballot because the time and resources involved would exceed our measurement of importance. The downside is that we will vote on those issues anyway, even though we don't have adequate information.

From a clinical perspective, we see asymmetric information used to convince a patient to have a procedure where if they had all the information they may choose not to. In these situations, the healthcare provider may provide all the information, but they can phrase their words in a way that may overwhelm a patient, and patients are normally so intimidated by their physicians that they will not question their recommendations. From an economic perspective, a solution to this asymmetry might be to increase the physician's compensation to get a more detailed explanation of the patient's symptoms and treatment options.

This circles back to our earlier discussion of Bartlett's *blind-date principle*. Think about the last movie that you went to see. I suspect you did a great deal of research on it. You looked up the actors and actresses, saw the trailer, and even read some reviews from other viewers. And this is for a movie that might cost you $10 to see. How about purchasing a car? Nowadays, you don't necessarily have to rely on what the salesperson tells you. You could go look up the value in the *Kelley Blue Book and* shop on the internet to dozens of other dealerships or even wholesalers online. You can research gas mileage and repair costs and reliability and safety, and again, you can read all kinds of reviews from other customers who have purchased and owned that vehicle. But how much research do we do on a blind date? In the prior two examples, we have dealt with the problem of asymmetry of information by doing our own research and balancing the information we got from the vendor with information we were able to find independently. But when we're going on a blind date, that's not what usually happens. A friend may say to us "He (or she) is really nice and loves animals and enjoys quiet walks on the beach." And that may be all the information we get. We don't do background checks to whether the person has a criminal record. Think about it, this could be the best or the worst night of your life, and we spend less time researching relevant information that we do going to the movies or purchasing a vehicle. The general rule is this: we almost always make our decisions with partial and inaccurate information.

So, what we do about that? Well, the key step is to simply recognize that this condition exists. We should know most of the information that we get regarding the decisions that we need to make is asymmetrical in one form or another. And depending on how critical the outcome of that decision will be, may be measured by risk and utility, we must be sure to allocate whatever resources are necessary to ensure the most positive outcome.

The Law of Diminishing Returns

We also must consider the law of diminishing returns. In general, this is that point on the graph where the cost of the information, whether in dollars or human capital or time, exceeds the value or the benefits that we receive. The best example of this I have seen has to do with collections within a healthcare organization. Based on which study you read, on average, it costs a healthcare provider about 14% to collect the money owed to them for the services and procedures that they perform on a given patient population. And that 14% will usually result in a collection of 95% to 96% of the monies that are owed. In one study; the researcher estimated that it would cost another 20% to 25% to collect the remaining 5% not collected on the first cycle. In this case, the cost of collecting exceeds the value of the collections. Actually, that sounds like a pretty good strategy to me if you are a payer.

We also see this sometimes when trying to determine the appropriate number of FTE employees per provider, particularly in physician practices. There areas benchmark data that will provide this type of information; however, it is sometimes difficult to apply in variable situations because we simply don't have enough information to determine how or why any other given organization's ratio is what it is. For example, if we increase the number of workers, let's say adding a physician or nonphysician practitioner, without increasing the workspace, then we will not see an equitable return on that investment. Even though we have an additional worker, we do not have the resources for that worker to generate revenue. I can't remember who said it, but sometimes the gain is simply not worth the pain.

I think, to some degree, we can interpret this as a way of differentiating between good and bad information as well. There's no question that there is some cost for good information. But the cost for bad information can sometimes be more. Particularly when there is a high utility factor tied to the outcomes of our decisions.

Rational Decision Making

Perhaps the best definition I have seen on rational decision-making was in a Hubspot blog entry called "Rational Decision Making: The 7 Step Process for Making Logical Decisions," written by Clifford Chi:

> Rational decision-making leverages objective data, logic, and analysis instead of subjectivity and intuition to help solve a problem or achieve a goal. It's a step-by-step model that helps you identify a problem, pick a solution between multiple alternatives, and find an answer.

Shortly, I am going to go over the steps involved in rational decision-making, and while this is a broad concept, it does go to the heart of the decision-making model. When considering this, I think we must ask ourselves an important question. Do the ends justify the means or do the ends justify the rationalization? In management, decisions must be both rational and legal. Here's an example. Let's say you live in some urban community and you working a 9 to 5 job like the majority of everyone else within that community. When 5 o'clock comes around, everybody leaves to go home. If everyone gets onto the highway, the highway quickly becomes clogged and a traffic jam ensues. So, people get off at the exits to get onto surface or secondary roads. But if everybody does that, soon the highway becomes unclogged and the traffic jams are on the secondary roads. When that happens, everyone moves from the secondary roads back to the highway and… You can see what happens moving forward.

There are some problems with choosing rationality when it comes to decision-making. The first is that we simply have a finite capacity to process information and understand data. Thirty years ago, my biggest problem was not being able to get access to enough information. Today, the problem is that there is too much information, and it is sometimes nearly impossible to sort through it all to determine what's usable and what's not. Human beings simply have a finite capacity when it comes to solving complex problems and processing all the information that might be available.

Another problem has to do with limits on the amount of time we have to solve problems. There is this issue that people have that I call "paralysis of analysis." This is where we are so caught up in wanting to get more and more information before making a decision that we simply become paralyzed and run out of time. I know this has happened to me on a number of occasions. I get to where I'm ready to make the decision, and then I think, "If I just had one more piece of data or one more block of information or one more article." And I run out of time. The other problem has to do with the limitations on the amount of information that we might be able to obtain or to filter. It's not just the quantity of information, but it's the quality of that information as well. And the accuracy of the data and the potential asymmetry based on the source.

Simple vs. Complex Systems

In my opinion, the most important consideration with respect to positive outcomes has to do with the state of the system. In general, there are two types: a simple and a complex system. Often, people will confuse 'complex' with 'complicated,' and there is a significant difference. In fact, a complicated system is just a more involved simple system. Here's an example: in a typical game of chess, if each player makes 40 moves in total, there are 10 to the 120th power possible combinations of moves. Does this make chess complicated or complex? It makes it complicated. What makes chess complex is the fact that there's more than one player. A complicated system is still pretty predictable, but that is not always true in a complex system. Another example has to do with vehicular travel. My van is a complicated piece of equipment. There are a lot of moving parts, and how it works is simply beyond my comprehension. But I could learn, and then I could fix it. Traffic is a complex system. Why? Because there are so many different drivers. So, the substantial difference between complex and simple systems is the number of actors or players or participants involved. Below is a great illustration of the complexity of the leased PPO network industry, as designed and published by the American Medical Association:

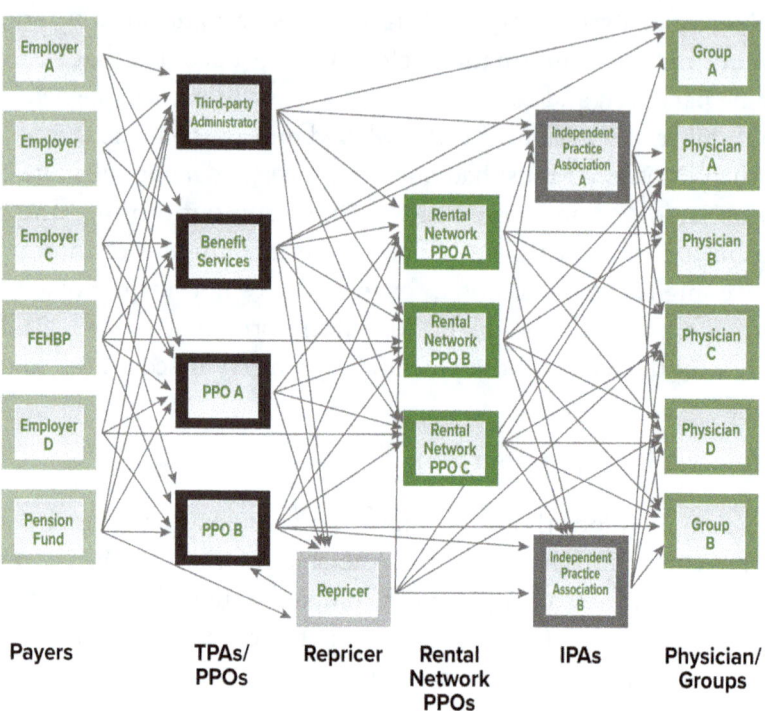

Figure 3.1 The Leased PPO Network Industry

This certainly illustrates the multitude of interactions going on within just a single payment model, so imagine the complexity of the complexities involved with just third-party payers.

From the standpoint of decision-making, most of us have been taught canonical methods that rely upon uncertainty and risk in a strongly linear way. Interestingly enough, complex systems also depend upon uncertainty and risk, but there are usually many more uncertainties than in a simple system. To better make this point, let's look at how decisions might be made in simple systems. Again, we are going to assess this as a component of rational decision theory. While there are many models out there, I like to stick to a four-step process that has worked successfully for me in the past.

Rational Decision Theory

As discussed above, we base this on three major concepts: uncertainty, risk, and utility. The four steps to decision-making using this model are as follows:

1. Imagine future states or conditions.
2. Determine the payoff or the consequence of each state.
3. Model the uncertainty and predictions of future events.
4. Calculate expected value (ROI).

Remember, this works well in simple linear systems because they are quite predictable and not as well in complex or nonlinear systems, which are far less predictable. I will talk more about decision-making models for complex systems later.

Let's pull from a real-life example. I have a small practice (three physicians) that is investigating whether to get an EHR system.

Imagine Future States

The first step for them is to imagine future states or conditions. They determine there are three potential future states. The first is that they remain a small practice without any expectations for growth or major change. In this case, they would want to select an online system that did not require any hardware or software maintenance. These systems are normally much less expensive, but they are not scalable. The second potential future is that the practice is going to grow, adding more physicians and/or nonphysician practitioners. If this is the case, then the EHR system might have to be a client/server-based application that would require them to purchase hardware and software. These are normally templated systems that will allow the practice to model the EHR around different specialties and services. They are also scalable but significantly more expensive. The third future that they imagine was that they were either going to be purchased or merged into a large organization like a bigger practice or hospital, or maybe even just close. For this future state, the best decision would be to delay the purchase altogether.

Determine Payoff

Step two is to determine the payoff for each future state. For the first state, where they remain a small practice, if they were to have engaged a vendor that provided the EHR as a software as a service (SaaS), and they stayed small, it would be a good payoff. But if they grew, adding physicians and/or nonphysician practitioners, requiring them to replace that EHR with a more complex system then it would've been a bad payoff. If they predicted that they would grow and purchase a system based on that expectation and they did grow, that would be a good payoff. But, in this state, if they stayed small and did not experience any growth, they would've overpaid for a system that was more than what they needed. That would've been a bad payoff. The third future state predicted that their practice was going to close or merge or be absorbed soon. If this panned out, then delaying the decision would be a good payoff. But, if it didn't, and they had to continuing practice for whatever reason, then they would be farther behind the eight ball when it came to integration of important technology, resulting in a bad payoff.

Modeling Uncertainty

The third step involves doing some quantitative predictions. In many cases, we do our best to guess what the outcomes might be. This is particularly true when we don't have a lot of prior experience or established data upon which to rely. So, for the purposes of this example, we are going to keep it simple. There is an old Danish proverb that statisticians and economists love: "It's hard to make predictions, especially about the future." In our example, for the future state of staying small, the team predicted there was an 80% probability that would happen and a 20% probability that some other future might occur. When it came to a small practice that might grow, they said there was a 65% probability that they would grow and a 35% probability that they would stay small. When it came to merging or closing, they predicted an 80% probability they would merge and close and a 20% probability that they would continue and practice.

It is important here not to confuse the difference between uncertainty and ambiguity. In project management for example, one might use a Gantt chart to estimate the amount of time it will take for processes to complete. In most cases, this is a best guess model. Rather than relying upon a single point estimate, the time to completion is a range. For example, 1 to 3 days, or 3 to 4 weeks. This is a quantifiable *uncertainty*, even though we may not have all the information necessary to derive some exact point estimate. Ambiguity is more complex, as it involves a knowledge of the options available. So, in this case, the practice came up with three potential future states or options. For each of these options, they modeled the uncertainty using some probabilistic method, even though they knew going into it that their estimates would not be exact. Hence the uncertainty. The ambiguity is whether there are more than three options. Often, different stakeholders or players can have different perspectives not only on the problem but on the solution or potential solutions as well. This is what makes ambiguity more complex than uncertainty. If you have several players, and each one has a different perspective, then when you combine those, you have a group ambiguity that is even greater than any single individual.

Calculating Expected Value

The fourth and final step is to calculate the expected value, or the return on investment, for each of the options or futures in the example. Mathematically speaking, we calculate the expected value as the sum of all the possible values multiplied by the probability of its occurrence. For example, the cost of engaging a vendor for an EHR as a software as a service (SaaS) model, as opposed to some other option. In this case, we would multiply the cost of the service times 80%, which is the probability of that future state existing, and then add that to the cost of an alternative system multiplied by the 20% probability that that future state would exist. My experience is that decision trees are the best tools for calculating these expected values.

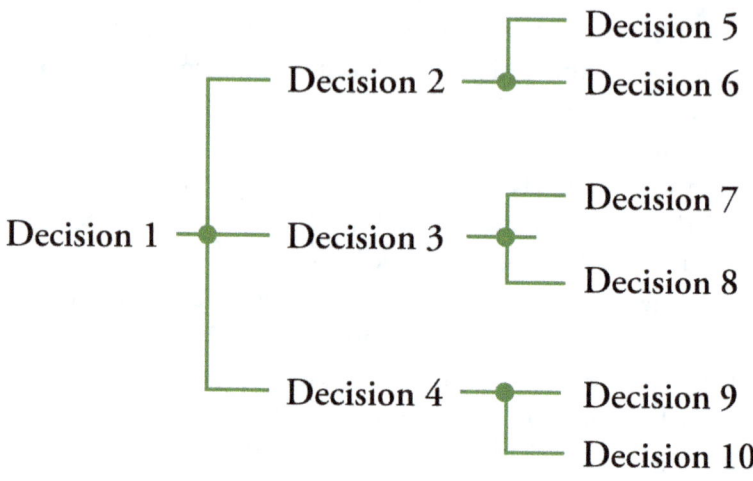

Figure 3.2 Decision Tree

As shown in the diagram above, it's simply a matter of quantifying the value for each of the nodes for our decision tree. One of the most famous decision trees is one called "Pascal's Wager" and of note is how applicable this is in complex as well as simple systems. In fact, when I talk about complex systems later, I will show you an example of using Pascal's Wager in those situations.

Blaise Pascal was 17th century French mathematician and physicist. As was the norm in those days, mathematicians were also philosophers and theologians. Considered the father of probability theory, he had this opinion that people would bet their lives on the belief that either God existed, or God did not exist. And from a purely probabilistic standpoint, Pascal opined that a rational person would always live their lives as though God did exist. Using a decision tree, it looks like the following:

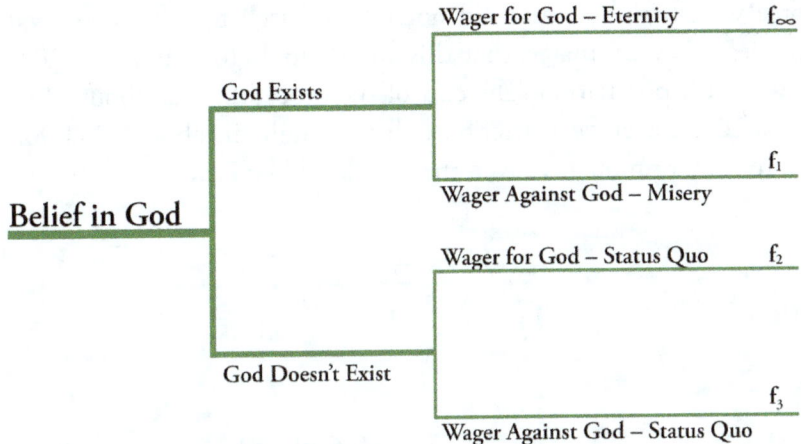

FIGURE 3.3 Pascal's Wager

The argument goes like this: either there is a God or there isn't a God. If God does exist and you live your life as though God exists, then the reward is eternal, or in this case infinite. As Pascal put it, "Our proposition is of infinite force." If God does exist, and you live your life as though there isn't a God, or as Pascal put it, wager against God, it is a life of misery. The second option is that God doesn't exist. If God doesn't exist and you live your life as though God does exist, then Pascal determined it to be status quo. While you may live a good life, there is no different material consequences than if you don't. And if you live your life as though there isn't a God and in fact God does not exist, then again, he opined, it would be the status quo.

— E(wager for God) = $\infty * p + f_1 * (1 - p) = \infty$

— E(wager against God) = $f_2 * p + f_3 * (1 - p) = f_n$

FIGURE 3.4 Pascal's Wager

Using a probability calculation as indicated above, Pascal concluded that, "The smart gambler always wagers on God."

45

Let's look at a simple expected value calculation on a real problem that involved a neurology and pain management practice in the southeastern United States. This group had developed a treatment for people with whiplash that did not respond well to other conservative therapies. They estimated that this would apply to only about 10% of the whiplash population. The cost of the procedure was about $15,000, but based on average collections, they brought in about $30,000. So, the profit margin on any given the case would be 2:1.

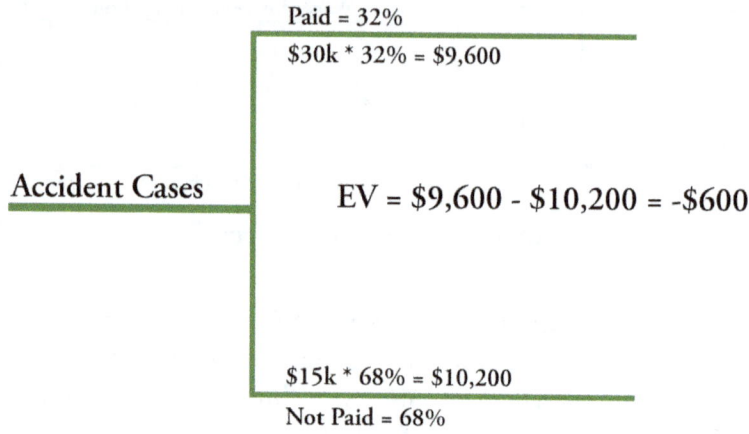

FIGURE 3.5 Accident cases

A little research showed that, in these types of cases and in this particular state, physicians were paid for these services about one-third of the time and two-thirds of the time they weren't. So, we multiply the $30,000, which is what they would be paid, times 32%, which represented the percent of time that they could expect to be paid for this procedure. This means that, on average, they would generate $9,600 in payments. Next, we look at the costs involved. They estimated their hard cost was about $15,000 per case. If paid 32% of the time, then 68% of the time they received no payment at all. So, we multiply the $15,000 times the 68%, and we get $10,200, which is the average cost per case. Let's sum them up. On average, they collect $9,600 and on average it cost $10,200, which means that over some given period, they will lose $600 on each case. Makes the decision simple.

I use this in my business all the time. Let's say I am working on a post audit extrapolation case. The practice had an audit done and the extrapolated estimated overpayment amount is $1 million. Let's say that I charge them $10,000 to do an analysis and deliver a report. I predict that there is a 10% probability we will get the extrapolation thrown out. That means that there's a 90% probability that we won't. So, we multiply the million dollars times 10% and we get $100,000. Then we multiply the cost of $10,000 times 90%, we get -$9,000. When we sum these together, we get an expected value of $91,000. So, unless the probability of us winning gets down to the 1% range, it's usually worth it to spend $10,000 to challenge the extrapolation.

This system that we have been discussing, this model, if you will, works better in simple systems. Let's spend a few minutes talking about complex systems. By definition, a complex system is a system composed of interconnected parts that exhibit one or more properties that are not obvious from the properties of the individual parts. Complex systems are usually quite diverse as well as interdependent, yet at the same time connected and highly adaptive. Three key characteristics of a complex system are:

1. They are unpredictable.
2. They produce large events.
3. They are very robust.

The economy, for example, is a complex system. There are many moving parts and many players, and many stakeholders all interconnected. The problem with trying to predict the outcome of a complex system is that you first must be able to predict the behavior of each of the individual stakeholders. I imagine all of us remember the financial crisis of 2008. Banks were going belly up, the housing market was crashing and burning, retirement accounts and pensions were in the toilet, and it was all doom and gloom. While I am hesitant to say that this wasn't predictable, because there are those that did predict this was going to happen at some point, it did produce an exceptionally large event and ultimately showed how robust our economy really is. Amid the crisis, people still had jobs and still had places to live and still had food to eat. I'm not trying to minimize how devastating the impact was for many people, I'm just trying to point to the fact that the economy as a system survived. We can also go back and look at the Deepwater Horizon accident that we discussed earlier. Hundreds of millions of gallons of crude oil dumped into the Gulf of Mexico resulted in the utter extinction of many species and the near extinction of others. And again, without minimizing the devastating impact that this had, we still have a Gulf of Mexico and we still have marine life and plant life and animal life and, despite all that, the coastal economy survived.

We can see the same impact within our own industry. When Congress finally passed the ACA, I would venture to say a sizable portion of it that resulted in the inability to predict the outcome within the insurance markets. Today, looking back, I believe we can validate the truth behind that concern. Because of the complexity of government, we are still trying to analyze the impact of this massive legislative change to the healthcare system. In addition to being unpredictable, it is hard to argue that it produced a large event. And it's also hard to argue against the robustness of the healthcare system. Because even though there were many negative impacts, we still have a healthcare system and patients are still seeing doctors and procedures are still going on, etc. This is a bit of a two-edged sword. The fact that it is a complex system means that it is unlikely it will fail, while making business and management decisions more difficult and less predictable.

Game Theory

If canonical decision theory does not work well in complex systems, then what should/do we do? There are four reasons why canonical decision theory does not apply in complex systems.

1. The model doesn't consider the behavior of other interested actors.
2. The model translates complexity into uncertainty.

3. The model is all exploitation.
4. The model focuses on a single outcome, not on system properties like connectedness, interdependence, diversity, and rates of learning and selection.

Let's look at these one at a time.

The Model Doesn't Consider the Behavior of Other Interested Actors

I think we've already described this in the description of a complex system itself. Using our EHR example, it would be simple to make a decision on the purchase of a system if the purchase only impacted one person or maybe one department or team. But that is simply not the case. EHR systems have tentacles that reach out to every aspect of the organization. The vendor has their own set of uncertainties, which include training, hardware integration, and implementation schedules. The physicians have their own set of uncertainties, which might include concerns over productivity, transformation of documentation, and coding paradigms. Administration has its own uncertainties, which involve timing and costs. IT has its own uncertainties around security. And the staff have their own set of uncertainties, which might include training and threats to their jobs. In essence, trying to bundle all the uncertainties under one distribution is all but impossible.

Game theory is an excellent tool for strategic decision-making and complex systems. But it is not a panacea for poor management skills. From the perspective of decision-making, they designed game theory for situations where two or more players drive the decisions. The game rock, paper, scissors is an excellent example. Think about it. If you knew that your opponent would throw paper every single time, then you would throw scissors every single time. But you don't. In fact, there are nine possible responses within a game of rock, paper, scissors and not knowing which of the three your opponent will present requires, by definition, complex decision-making skills. Maybe your opponent tells you that they are going to throw paper. Do you believe them? Do you have history with that person? Have they been dishonest with you in the past?

In these sorts of situations, your decisions become dependent on the decisions of others. In this example, each player needs to consider all the possible strategies of the other players in order to determine the decision that gives him/her the best payoff. It's impossible to find the perfect solution, so we shoot for the optimal solution instead. Within game theory, the primary goal is to find an equilibrium amongst the players, and in game theory this is the Nash equilibrium. The Nash equilibrium maintains its focus on rivalries with mutual gain. It is a set of mixed strategies for finite noncooperative games between two or more players whereby no player can improve his or her payoff by changing their strategy.

A *Nash equilibrium* occurs when each player knows what the other players strategy is and no one player has an incentive to change their strategy for personal gain. Let's look how this might apply to us in the healthcare field by looking at our relationship with the payers. Raise your hand if this has ever happened to you. You submit a claim for some procedures or services, and you be getting paid on a regular basis by some given payer. Then, one day, the claim gets denied and assigned some specific reason and/or remark code. So, you research it, make changes that are necessary and resubmit the claim and this time you get paid. And that goes on for a while until you get another denial for another reason and you must figure out how to clean that up and submit the claims again. And the cycle continues *ad nauseum*. Because, under most circumstances, we do not have a Nash equilibrium with the payers. I would posit that the payer, in fact, is incentivized to change their audit strategy for personal gain. It's not evil, it's just business. We can say that each player strategy is an optimal response based on the anticipated rational strategy of the other player(s) in the game.

The most classic example of game theory is what's called the prisoner's dilemma. The graphic below illustrates the scenario.

	Prisoner B Stays Silent	**Prisoner B Betrays**
Prisoner A Stays Silent	*Each serves 6 months*	*Prisoner A: 10 years* *Prisoner B: goes free*
Prisoner A Betrays	*Prisoner A: goes free* *Prisoner B: 10 years*	*Each serves 5 years*

TABLE 3.1 Prisoner's dilemma

Let's say that I am at a conference and I meet some guy there, and we decide we're going out to get dinner somewhere. On our way out of the hotel, we see this beautiful Aston Martin Vulcan parked out front. This is a $2 million car. We sneak the keys away from the valet, we jump in, and we steal it. We're flying down the road and end up having an accident. By the time the police get there, we are both sitting on the curb next to the car. As is common in investigations of this type, the police separate us and question us individually. What they want to know is who is driving the car. To incentivize us to talk, we are both offered a deal.

If we both stay quiet and don't rat on each other, we will each spend six months in jail. But if one of us rats on the other, before the other rats first, the first one will go free and the second one will get ten years. So, if I rat out my friend first, I go free and he gets ten years. But if he rats me out first, he goes free and I get ten years. If we both ran at each other out at the same time, we both get five years. So, the clock is ticking. In this model, each prisoner receives the greatest reward if they betray the other, but only if the other does not betray them. So hopefully, you can see here that knowing the other person strategy is critical for each of us to receive the optimal reward. It's important to note that the optimal reward is not always the best reward. In this scenario, my decision would be based on how well I knew the other person, and how well I could trust them to stay quiet.

I remember some time ago that there was a lot of talk about the importance of the medical home. A patient-centered philosophy that drives primary care excellence, the term "patient centered" is used in the sense that the patients and the families are intimately involved in the decisions that are made for treatment, and that the providers respect those patients needs and preferences. It also ensures that there is significant effort put toward education and support for treatment decisions. The medical home also involves more comprehensive care, or a holistic approach. The philosophy is to treat the whole person, which includes all physical, mental, and emotional needs. The third feature of the medical home is accessibility. Patients should have shorter waiting times and access to after hour care, including telephonic care around the clock.

One of the key features of a medical home is coordination of care, something that is sorely lacking in our healthcare system today. This means that all the providers involved in the care of the patient are aware of all the treatments and procedures and medications associated with that patient. From my own personal experience, I have seen many organizations claim to embrace the medical home philosophy but, in fact, are no different than any other organization. From a financial perspective, the idea of economic reward comes from savings rather than volume. Right now, everyone is competing for a finite amount of dollars to pay for services and procedures for any given patient population. So, if you want to make more, you must do more. The problem is, if you do more and so does everyone else, it diminishes the value per unit of service. And when that happens, you must do even more to make more and that diminishes the value per unit of service. I will stop now because I'm confident that you're getting the big picture here.

So, why did the medical home fizzle out? Let's approach this from the idea of the prisoner's dilemma.

	They base on volume	They base on outcomes
I base on volume	*Equal cost* *Equal revenue* *Inefficient care*	*I thrive* *They suffer* *Efficient care*
I base on outcomes	*I suffer* *They thrive* *Inefficient care*	*Equal cost* *Equal revenue* *Efficient Care*

TABLE 3.2 Outcomes versus volume dilemma

Let's say that I decide to embrace the medical home philosophy, meaning that my revenue will be based more on outcomes than volume. In order for this to work, all the other physicians within some given geographic boundary also have to embrace the medical home philosophy, because if they don't, then I will be competing on uneven ground against those who are still diminishing the pie through volumetric based care. In that scenario, I suffer, they thrive, and the result is inefficient care. If everyone else adopts the medical home philosophy, and I don't, I thrive, they suffer, and we have inefficient care. If everyone maintains the status quo and focuses on the volume of care rather than outcomes, we have equal cost, equal revenue, and inefficient care. The problem is getting everyone to agree to take a risk with this new model. I can't get four physicians to agree on a strategic plan, much less an entire community of physicians to agree to an economic model. So, in this scenario, each physician receives the greatest reward if they continue to base their revenue on volume, but only if the other physicians don't. So, what happens? Nothing changes. It's my opinion that if you want treatment models like medical home to succeed, legislation is needed to make it a requirement.

The Model Translates Complexity into Uncertainty

As we have seen, complex systems are very dependent upon other actors within the system and, as such, we often confuse complexity with uncertainty. Complexity deals with the interactions and interrelationships between actors and entities. Uncertainty deals with the predictive probabilities for each of those interactions or inter-relationships. As an example, let's go back to the idea of getting an EHR for your organization. The complexity issue deals with the interrelationships between the parties: the vendor, the physicians, the administration, billing and coding, IT, end users, etc. Where the confusion often lies is that we look at this complexity and define it as not just uncertainty but as one uncertainty. We think that we can model this as though each of these interrelationships are terminally connected to some single outcome; they are not. There is the uncertainty curve of training, which involves the vendor and the staff. And each of these have their own uncertainty distributions. As stated, the vendor may see training successfully completed in six months, while the real training takes closer to a year. How do you handle the loss of productivity or the transition issues during that additional non-scheduled time? And what about acceptance? The physician's will have their own distribution of uncertainty, which will likely be different than the staff (say, front and back office) and maybe IT is going to have an implementation schedule that doesn't jive with the implementation schedule projected by the vendor or required by administration.

The solution to this is to carefully look at each connection in the relationships, define each actor or entity's role and work with them to define their needs, expectations, and objections. When complete, it becomes only a matter of properly combining and parsing those uncertainties into a model that fits within the complexity of the organization.

The Model is all Exploitation

What this means is that in a simple, linear system, the model tends to be based on tradition and traditional expectations. It exploits, if you will, existing models and comes to rely on their successes and failures. Again, in linear systems, this is often good enough, but in complex systems, it is not. The counteraction to exploitation is to look at the issue from a more Bayesian approach. Without getting into all the math involved from a formal perspective, Bayesian probability uses a conditional component that describes the probability of an event occurring based on the presence of some other event having occurred. For example, when we looked at the issue of mammograms, we were interested not in just the probability that a women had breast cancer or the probability that she had a positive mammogram, but rather the probability that she had breast cancer *given* the fact that she did have a positive mammogram. We are not necessarily interested in whether a venture will fail, *per se*, but whether the venture will fail *given* that some other factor or event has already occurred or is present. Using this approach, we can move from exploitation to a more non-linear model. The model focuses on a single outcome, not on system properties like connectedness, interdependence, diversity, rates of learning, and selection.

Ready, Aim, Fire

Quite often, the problem with decision making is really in the execution. So often, decisions are made but never implemented, or they are implemented before they are made (I will explain that in a moment). There are lots of reasons for this and much is written in the literature about a 'failure to launch,' but, in my experience, it all boils down to one problem: a paralysis of analysis or the rapid fire method, both resulting from a fear of making the wrong decision. Let's look at the three iterations of this model:

1. Ready, ready, ready, ready . . .
2. Ready, aim, ready, aim, ready, aim . . .
3. Fire, fire, fire, fire, fire . . .

Ready, Ready, Ready, Ready . . .

Simply put, this first case is about too much planning and too little doing. Often, we find ourselves in the situation of not being able to plan through the decision process because we failed to define the problem in the first place. For example, on one engagement, I was working with the client on building a fee schedule that would be reasonable and effective for all payers. This would have involved looking at peer benchmarks, modeling RVUs and conversion factors, considering payments from other payers, being sensitive to the community's needs, etc. But we never got that far. The practice was stuck in the planning phase, arguing about the importance of the fee schedule, how patients and payers might receive it, whether they would be judged either non-competitive or too competitive, etc. They never got to the point of even conducting research or benchmarking their existing fees to see where they stood in both their local community as well as a broader market view. Nope. They got stuck in the planning phase; they were unable to even define the problem or their goals and objectives.

Ready, Aim, Ready, Aim . . .

The next and perhaps most prevalent issue I have encountered is this problem with failure to launch. This is where they create a plan and conduct research, but they don't pull the trigger. This paralysis of analysis is always looking for one more datum point or one more piece of information of just a little more evidence to support the case. I remember working with a practice considering adding another provider. We created a primary research project where we were looking at visits per unit of time and work RVUs per visit for the existing docs to see how readily they could support another physician, or whether it would be a better idea to get a PA or NP instead. The decision matrix was a bit complex because, in addition to looking at actual time/schedule/work RVU-type data, we also had to consider community buy-in (which required some questionnaires) as well as other hard data, like licensing restrictions and payer requirements. We looked at 90 days of patient visits in our forward approach, as planned, but before making the decision, leadership wanted to look at one more months' worth of data. And after that, it was another month and then another month . . . ready, aim, ready, aim, ready, aim! It took just over a year to finally come to a decision and, lo and behold, it was the same decision supported at the 90-day point.

Analysis paralysis, or over thinking, is a big problem within a lot of organizations for whom I have conducted analyses. These may have been for operational efficiencies, capital improvement, physician recruitment, and even the introduction of new technologies. In all cases, the inability to make a decision was costly; perhaps more costly, in some cases, than making the wrong decision. At some point, someone has to flick the switch. Sometimes, the problem is more simple than complex. Sometimes, it's just that someone (or everyone) is afraid to make a decision for fear of getting it wrong. There are couple of ways to attack this issue. One is to set a drop-dead date and *stick to it*. Another is to just admit that, at some point, more data is not going to help. This is where we get into an understanding of the law of diminishing returns.

Fire, Fire, Fire

The last, but certainly not the least destructive, perturbation is the concept of just throwing things against the wall and hoping something sticks. The reason that this is so potentially destructive is that wrong decisions (many of them) can be quite costly, particularly in areas of high criticality. Hiring a bunch of docs and finding out that didn't fix the problem is quite costly. Putting up a new building or adding onto an existing one, only to find out that flow rather than space was the problem, can be more costly. Trying out new products without testing can result in reductions in quality, which has its own costly liabilities.

I was brought into one large organization that had committed to a significant reduction in costs over a short period (less than a year) and asked for my assistance. I told them that there was no way to do this responsibly within the time constraints. So, they wanted to know the irresponsible way, which was to just start cutting staff: a dangerous move without a complex and comprehensive impact analysis. And that's what they did, and the results were near catastrophic. Remaining staff were often so overburdened that they left. The practice saw increases in errors and mistakes. Continuity of care suffered, as did quality, and the result was a more severe impact on revenue than on costs. In the end, they hired a new CEO, but getting back to baseline was about as difficult as starting over. The moral of the story? Sometimes no decision is better than a bad decision, as it is certainly counterproductive to confuse movement with progress.

To Sum Up . . .

Decision-making takes on many forms. Not every decision is complex. In fact, not every decision is difficult to make. More times than not, the decisions we make result in a positive outcome. My position is that we should quantify, and measure as much as makes sense to ensure that in more difficult and complex decisions, we can increase the likelihood of a positive outcome. We will never be anything like perfect decision-makers, but we can become optimal decision-makers.

Let's say that you have an employee that shows up late, leaves early, and doesn't do his work when he is there. You won't have to form a committee or research the internet to find data to support the options that you have. In most cases, the person is fired. A mosquito lands on your arm. You don't need to take a picture of it and submit it to some website for an entomologist to identify it before you find a solution. You swat it. You wake up at 3 o'clock in the morning, and your house is on fire. You don't start calculating the combustion rate of your furniture, you run. Wouldn't it be nice if all our decisions were that black-and-white? But they are not. For evidence-based decision-making,

I am proposing that we take our practical problems, convert them to analytical problems, find an analytical solution, and then convert those back to practical solutions.

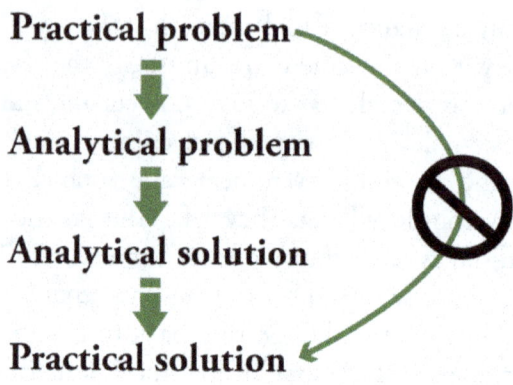

FIGURE 3.6 Practical problem to practical solution flow

So, what are the pitfalls of anecdotal thinking? Particularly when dealing with a higher order of problems that require a more complex approach to decision making? The first is a failure to observe. We have all seen this happen, and in fact, I have been guilty of this myself. I remember my first interim CEO position at a mid-size hospital. In my first week, I gathered all the department heads, directors, and VPs together like they were my minions or something like that. Then, I proceeded to tell them all the fabulous changes I had in mind even though, at that time, I didn't have a clue about how the organization worked. I just assumed that, because my ideas worked somewhere in the past, they would work here as well. I assumed that I knew what their problems, issues, and shortcomings were without taking the time to research it myself or consult with those in the know.

The second is a failure to plan. Let's say that I do some investigating. I gather evidence and determine where there are processes to improve or even eliminate. But rather than sit down and plan out some strategy, I just dive headfirst into trying to apply a fix without have first gone through the proper process. A cause-and-effect analysis would have been a better idea. Or simulating the fix first to see what unexpected consequences might arise. Failure to plan happens when we assume how to fix a problem without first finding out what is causing it.

Finally, there is the failure to validate. This is where we assume that the action taken to fix the problem has worked without measuring to see if it is really doing what we wanted or expected. For example, let's say we make a change to the scheduling model for one of our clinics or for a department. We wait a month and then cascade the change to all the other clinics or departments. But wait! It would be helpful to know whether that change resulted in a positive or negative outcome. Because if it was negative, then why in the world would we want to impose it on anyone else? It is my opinion that this is the most overlooked step in modeling change: failure to measure the outcomes of change to evaluate its effectiveness.

CHAPTER 4
It's All About the Evidence

I would like to begin this section with an example of how critical thinking and the use of analytics can play a huge and influential role in science and society. Often, we tend to stay focused on the small picture, and by that I mean our own issues as they relate to us and our organizations. But there are big-picture issues that tend to trickle down to our issues and impact us both professionally and personally.

Prior to 1980, the American Cancer Society recommended that women between the ages of 40 and 49 have a mammogram "if they or their mother or sisters had breast cancer." By May of 2003, the recommendation was that women aged 40 to 49 receive a screening mammogram every year. But something happened. A study was published in 2009 by the United States Preventive Services Task Force (USPSTF) in the *Annals of Internal Medicine* which, among other findings, concluded that screening mammograms for women in this age group carried a higher risk than a benefit. Much of the evidence supporting this conclusion was based on a Bayesian statistical analysis of the results of hundreds of thousands of tests done over more than a decade of time. The question that I find the most interesting is this: if a 40- to 49-year-old woman has a positive mammogram, what's the probability that she has breast cancer?

Let's look at some of the predicates to this study:

- 1% of women in their forties who participated in routine screening were diagnosed with breast cancer
- 80% of women who have breast cancer got a positive mammogram
- 9.6% of women in this age group who *did not* have breast cancer got a positive mammogram (false positive or FP)

Bayes' Rule looks like this:

$$P(A \text{ if } B) = \frac{P(A \text{ and } B)}{P(B)}$$
$$\Rightarrow P(A \text{ and } B) = P(A \text{ if } B)P(B)$$
$$P(A \text{ and } B) = P(B \text{ if } A)P(A)$$
$$\Rightarrow P(A \text{ if } B) = \frac{P(A \text{ and } B)}{P(B)} = \frac{P(B \text{ if } A)P(A)}{P(B)}$$
$$\Rightarrow P(A \text{ if } B) = \frac{P(B \text{ if } A)P(A)}{P(B)} \quad \text{<- Bayes Rule}$$

FIGURE 4.1 Bayes' Rule

In general, it says that the probability of some event occurring, given some other event also occurs, is equal to the probability of the second event occurring, given that the first event also occurred, times the probability the first event occurs, all divided by the probability that the second event occurs. So, again, we want to know the probability of a woman in her forties having breast cancer (first event) *given that* she received a positive mammogram (the second event). In our case, the formula would look like this:

$$P(\text{cancer if positive}) = \frac{P(\text{positive if cancer})P(\text{cancer})}{P(\text{positive})}$$

FIGURE 4.2 Mammogram cancer probability formula

It's All About the Evidence

Let's assume that 100,000 women between the age of 40 and 49 are selected from the population at random to have a screening mammogram. The workflow would look something like what we see below:

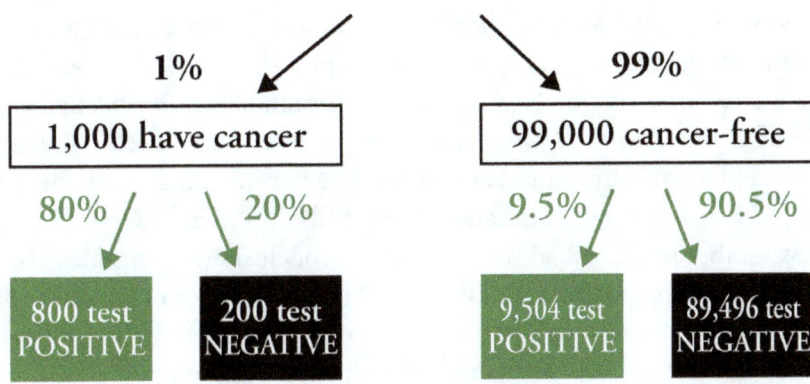

FIGURE 4.3 Mammogram probability tree

Of the 100,000 including in this study, 1% (or 1,000) truly have breast cancer, while 99% (99,000) do not. Of the 1,000 that do have cancer, approximately 80% (800) will report a positive mammogram (True Positive or TP), while 20%, or 200, will report a negative mammogram (False Negative, or FN). Of the 99,000 that are cancer-free, approximately 9.5% will report a positive mammogram (False Positive, or FP), while 89,496 will report a true negative (TN). This means that they did not have cancer and the mammogram was negative.

Now, let's work through the formula from above.

The chances that a woman has cancer if she has a positive mammogram is the TP times the number that have cancer, all divided by the number that tested positive overall. This latter figure would consist of those that had a TP (800) plus those that had a FP (9,504). The formula, then, would look something like this:

800/(800+9,504) = 7.8% of positive results have cancer

That's correct. The answer to the question is that, of all women who receive a positive mammogram, only 7.8% will be diagnosed cancer. If you are like me, you are probably a bit astounded. I will admit that, even though I have run these types of calculations many times in the past, I was a bit slack-jawed.

Now, it's good to note that this recommendation created a huge amount of controversy and the arguments went well beyond the economics, but it is good to at least understand that perspective. In April of 2015, *Health Affairs* magazine published an article entitled: "National Expenditure for False-Positive Mammograms and Breast Cancer Overdiagnoses Estimated at $4 Billion a Year." Wow. That's an eye-grabbing headline! One of their conclusions went like this: "Screening has the potential to save lives. However, the economic impact of false-positive mammography results and breast cancer overdiagnoses must be considered in the debate about the appropriate populations for screening." The cost? Based on a study of 702,154 women aged 40 to 49, "The average expenditures for each false-positive mammogram, invasive breast cancer, and ductal carcinoma *in situ* in the twelve months following diagnosis were $852, $51,837, and $12,369, respectively." In a study published in *Significance* magazine a couple of years ago, it put the average cost of a mammogram, due to the cost of false positives, at just over $35,000 each. That was quite a shock to both the medical and the insurance communities.

There were other negatives reported as well. For example, the health risk experienced from further workup and testing, including invasive diagnostic procedures. There was a great deal of personal stress and anxiety related to false positives and lost time at work due to both consequences. There were also medical injuries that occurred as a natural consequence of invasive testing performed to confirm the mammogram results. And while the results of this study may not do much to quell the controversy, the facts are the facts and should account for something.

In evidence-based medicine, healthcare providers engage in something called differential diagnosis. Differential diagnosis refers to the methods by which we consider the possible causes of a patient's clinical findings before making a final diagnosis and recommend treatment options. Critical thinking in respect to the process is, well, critical! According to a 2015 study published by the National Academies of Sciences, Engineering and Medicine, some 12 million people, or about 5% of adults who seek outpatient care, are misdiagnosed annually. The study goes on to say that these diagnostic errors "contribute to approximately 10% of patient deaths" and "account for 6% to 17% of adverse events in hospitals." In a 2017 study from Mayo Clinic published in the *Journal of Evaluation in Clinical Practice*, the authors reported that, of the patients that come to them for a second or third opinion, only 12% receive confirmation that the original diagnosis was complete and correct. This is one of the reasons that so many people now search their symptoms online looking for answers and confirmation for what the doctor has told them. In a study released in 2018, by the Pew Internet & American Life Project, 80% of internet users—or about 93 million Americans—have searched for a health-related topic online.

So, what's wrong with your organization? What I am asking is, where does it hurt? Whether using a *reductio ad absurdum* approach or subjecting your systems to a complete "physical exam," differential diagnosis for the business is no different than differential diagnosis for the patient. We begin, then, by measuring. A familiar pithy saying states that, "You can't manage what you can't measure." As you will learn here, it is my opinion that we can measure pretty much everything. If something is observable within the universe, it is measurable, and the more observable it is, the easier it is to measure. A famous saying in the field of benchmarking is, "If you don't value it, you won't change it."

Let's take some time here to talk about this idea of benchmarking. The origin of this term is quite interesting, but I will let you do an internet search on your own to read about it. For our purposes, we can go with *The Oxford Dictionary* definition: "evaluate or check (something) by comparison with a standard." So, to benchmark, we need at least two vectors or scalars. In mathematics, a *vector* is an object that has both a magnitude and a direction. Velocity is a perfect vector, as it has a speed (how fast is the object going) and a direction (is it heading toward me or away from me?). A *scalar* is described by its magnitude only and is more commonly found in the work we will do.

In any case, we can always refer to what we are looking at as a data point or a variable. The first variable is the one we are interested in researching, such as FTEs, collections, wait time, etc., and it comes from our own internal data. The second data point is some standard and that, in and of itself, can be a real problem. For example, if you are looking to benchmark your revenue per unique beneficiary, would you be comfortable comparing against the Medicare data? What if you don't accept Medicare patients or if your mix is quite small? Do you have any idea whether the standard is one that represents your goals and objectives? There are many private firms and organizations that sell benchmark data, and it is incumbent upon the manager to research the impact that asymmetrical information will have on their efforts and results.

Benchmarking can take on two primary faces: internal and external. In external benchmarking, we are comparing some aspect of our business (FTEs, RVUs, collections per patient, wait time, etc.) against some standard. In internal benchmarking, we are comparing that same aspect but against a goal or objective. For example, a standard metric for collections at time-of-visit is 62%, but you want to do better than that, so you set an "internal benchmark," which is your own goal, to 75%. You then track your collection percent against your goal to assess your progress (or lack of it). I am not necessarily a fan of external benchmarking because it requires us to accept as gospel that the standard is, in fact, a reasonable and righteous standard. We often must accept that without all the information necessary to make that determination. Quite often, I see benchmark data represented as point estimates, like 3.6 FTEs per provider, or 5,100 work RVUs per provider or collection ratio of 51% or A/R of 32 days.

This is a perfect time to talk about some of the problems that we have coming up with measuring point estimates. By far, the average is the most often referenced point estimate. If you remember back to junior high or high school math, to get the average you simply add up the value of all the data points and then divide by the number of data points. It's that simple. But unless the data are normally distributed, the average is not the best estimator. The other problem is that whenever we use a sample, we naturally introduce some degree of error. And just like with measuring variability, if we don't measure and account for the error, then we don't have a full picture of the data.

Chapter 5
Basic Statistics for the Healthcare Manager

The last thing that I want to do is turn this book into a classroom text on mathematics and statistics. But there are at least four concepts that every manager needs to understand if they are going to work with analytics and data. They are as follows:

1. *Measures of location*, also called *central tendency*. For our purposes, this will include the mean, the median, and the mode.
2. *Measures of variation or dispersion*. This will include the range, the standard deviation, and the interquartile range.
3. *Measures of error or estimation*. This will include measurements of standard error and confidence intervals.
4. *Measures of relationships*. This includes the covariance, correlation, and regression, and we will only lightly touch on this last topic.

Measures of Position and Central Tendency

The three measures that we mostly focus on are the average (or the mean), the median, and the mode. The *average (or mean)* is the most common measure that people tend to use, but it is also the most inappropriate metric in the types of distributions we encounter in healthcare. In general, a distribution is a visualization of what the data look like when plotted on a graph, and I will discuss this in much greater detail shortly. The mean adds up all the values in the set of numbers and then divides the sum by the number of data points. Here's a simple example:

Code	CF
99201	41.60
99202	80.44
99203	121.36
99204	214.80
99205	307.91
99211	22.12
99212	40.18
99213	81.04
99214	116.90
99215	181.50
Total	**1207.85**
Average	**120.79**

TABLE 5.1   Averaging example

In this case, the sum of the values is 1,207.85. We divide this by the count of 10 data points, and we get an average of 120.79. Simple stuff. The problem is that the mean is sensitive to outliers. Let's say that the 99204 code had a conversion factor of 607.91 rather than the 307.91. In that case, the mean would have been 150.79; significantly higher than the prior average.

The *median*, on the other hand, doesn't care what the values are in the cells, but measures their location first. Let's look at that same example, only this time, we will measure the median value. The first step is to sort the data in ascending order by the variable of interest; in this case, the CF. Then, we go to the middle cell in the list. The middle because that is what the median represents: the 50th percentile. When there are an odd number of data points, selecting the middle value is easy. But when there is an even number, we must take one more step. In this case, we would average the 5th and 6th cell, so 81.04 + 116.90 = 197.94. Then, dividing by 2, we get the median value of 98.97.

Code	CF
99201	41.60
99202	80.44
99203	121.36
99204	214.80
99205	307.91
99211	22.12
99212	40.18
99213	81.04
99214	116.90
99215	181.50
Total	1207.85
Median	98.97

TABLE 5.2   Median example

This is quite different from the average (mean) value of 120.79. This is typically the case in a right-skewed distribution; the mean is higher than the median. The other benefit is that the median is not as sensitive to outliers as the mean and, in some cases, not at all. Let's go back to our example where the fee for the 99205 is 607.91. In this case, because it does not affect the middle cells, the median is still 98.97.

Back in 2016, I was the statistical expert in fraud case, and I was testifying during the penalty phase of the trial. The government had conducted two extrapolation audits on the physician's two clinics and wanted the judge to include the results in the damage estimate: a total of nearly $6 million. A huge issue was that, for both audits, the data were terribly right skewed and both data sets included extremely high outliers. As a result, the average was nearly twice the median. The judge asked me to give him an example of how outliers impact the mean, while the median remained constant. Here's the example I gave him:

> A statistician walks into a bar carrying a pencil and a pad of paper. There are 100 residents in the bar, and he goes around and asks each one what their earnings were over the past 12 months. Because we had a fairly homogenous population, the data were normally distributed and as a result, the mean and the median were both equal to the same value; $36,226. A few minutes later, Bill Gates walked into the bar and ordered a beer. Now, on average, everyone was a millionaire. But the median remained the same.

Any time the data are skewed one way or the other, the median will almost always be the most optimal and robust measure of central tendency. The last measure I will mention here is the mode. The *mode* is the value that shows up the most. This is determined by sorting the frequency for the value of interest in either ascending or descending order. The value that has the highest frequency is the mode. Personally, I don't rely on this a lot unless there is some specific reason, such as estimating the central tendency of fees or payments in a given market.

Another measurement that you will likely see are *percentile* rankings. In fact, we have already worked with one: the median, which is nothing more than the 50th percentile. This means that half of the values are higher than the median and half are lower than the median. And lest we get confused, in a skewed database, this is not always true when it comes to the mean. The "percentile" is different from the "percentage" and represents the location of the data point compared to all the other data points. For example, the 75th percentile means that only 25% of values are higher, while 74% of values are lower. Same with the 90th percentile, only 10% of value are higher, while 89% are lower. There are a lot of data sets commercially available that use percentiles. And most will report quartiles, which is just a fancy way of saying the 25th, the 50th (median) and the 75th percentiles.

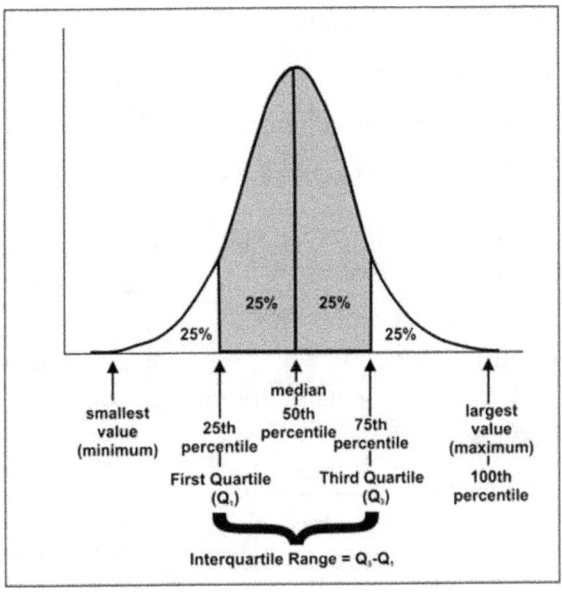

FIGURE 5.1   Bell curve distribution

For example, in physician compensation, we might look to pay a physician at the 75th percentile of their peers if they report at the 75th percentile for work RVUs or collections. Or maybe, we are trying to benchmark our front-end collection against other practices, and we want to be at the 90th percentile. In many of the large out-of-network class action cases where I worked as an expert, the payers would pay the physician at the 80th percentile of charges. Remember, the idea is that, with percentiles, we can compartmentalize the cells and therefore the values.

Here is an example of how we would use percentiles. The formula looks like this:

$$r = \frac{p(n+1)}{100} = I + D$$

Figure 5.2 Percentiles formula

where

P = the percentile you want to find

n = the total number of values

I = the integer part of the ranking

D = the decimal part of the ranking

This is an age distribution example, and we have 121 individual data points (n = 121). The 75th percentile for the age distribution, then, is (121*75/100) = 90.75, or around the 91st observation, when arranging the ages in ascending order. The 75th percentile of the ages is, therefore, 31 years. The 25th, 50th (median) are the 31st and 61st observations, respectively. It looks like this:

	Age	Frequency	Cumulative Frequency	
	21	6	6	
	22	16	22	The 31st observation falls in this group
25th percentile →	23	11	33 ←	
	24	9	42	
	25	17	59	The 61st observation falls in this group
50th percentile →	26	13	72 ←	
	27	6	78	
	28	5	83	
	29	4	87	
	30	3	90	The 91st observation falls in this group
75th percentile →	31	1	91 ←	
	32	4	95	
	33	3	98	
	34	2	100	
	35+	21	121	
	Total	121		

Figure 5.3 Age distribution

Variance

One of the big issues that we encounter, particularly from the standards that we use to benchmark, is that the variance or variability is often missing. I am of the opinion that a point estimate without variance is all but useless. Let's say that I go to a party, and I collect the age of each person there, and I calculate the average age as 40 years old. I call my wife, and I say, "Honey, I am so excited. I am at this party, and the average age here is 40 years old." That's great, but she has absolutely no idea what the group of people look like. For example, they could all be exactly 40 years old. That would give me an average age of 40 years old for sure. They might be between 30 and 50 years old or between 20 and 60 years old or between 10 and 70 years old. Without measuring variation, point estimates simply don't have any value. I heard a great joke once from this comedian. A police office stops him for doing 100 miles an hour in a 55 mile an hour zone. The officer asks him, "Did you know that the speed limit here is 55 miles per hour?" And the driver answers, "Well, I really didn't plan to be out driving for an hour."

Here's a fitting example of why measuring variance and visualizing data are so important. I was once engaged by a large group that was interested in hiring a physician and part of the contract included paying him a bonus for goodwill. That is, for him working to keep his existing patient population. The compensation part of the package was primarily based upon what his current collections look like. So, the physician prepared a control chart to show the stability of his collections over time. He measured his revenue as collections per RVU, and the charts that he produced showed an average of $79.19. Not bad, actually. This is what the chart that he produced looked like.

I asked for a monthly report of collections and RVUs over the past two years, a request that caused the physician to balk. But eventually, we received the data, and this is what it looked like over time.

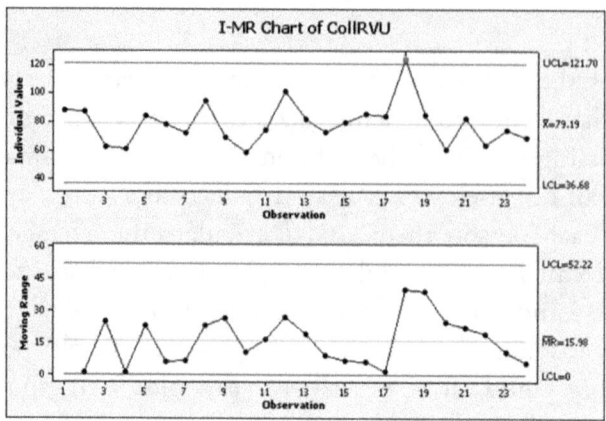

FIGURE 5.4   I-MR Chart of Collections and RVUs

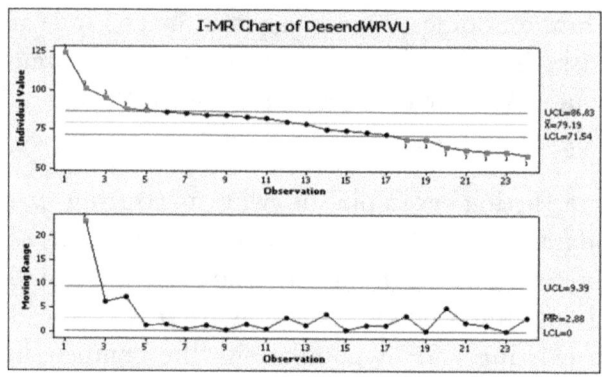

FIGURE 5.5   I-MR Chart of Collections and RVUs over two years

As you can see, it was a stark difference. In both analyses, the average remained precisely the same: $79.19 per RVU. The problem here with the first chart is that as the collections declined at about the same rate as the number of services, the average collection per RVU remained consistent. But without looking at the second analysis, we wouldn't have had any clue that this physician's business was on a steady decline. No wonder he wanted to sell his practice.

Basic Statistics for the Healthcare Manager

For the mean, we measure the *variance* using the *standard deviation*. We could spend an entire day on the statistics of variance, but for our purposes, I think I can explain it in much simpler terms. Let's go back to our table where we calculated the average and add a couple of columns.

The first two columns are the same: the code and the charge. In the third column (Delta), I subtracted the charge from the average. So, for 99201, I subtracted the average of 120.79 from 41.60 and got a result of -79.19. The most logical conclusion would be to just add all these numbers up to get the variance, but because we subtracted from the average, which is, for practical purposes, the halfway value, the sum of the deltas is zero. Makes perfect sense! Instead, we square the delta, which gives us a positive number, and then we add these up. Now we get the average of that squared difference (the variance) and take the square root, which in this case is 85.60.

Or, of course, you could just use one of the @stdev functions in Microsoft Excel (like I did). One way to better understand how this

Code	Charge	Delta	Variance
99201	41.60	(79.19)	6,271.06
99202	80.44	(40.35)	1,628.12
99203	121.36	0.57	0.32
99204	214.80	94.01	8,837.88
99205	307.91	187.12	35,013.89
99211	22.12	(98.67)	9,735.77
99212	40.18	(80.61)	6,497.97
99213	81.04	(39.75)	1,580.06
99214	116.90	(3.89)	15.13
99215	181.50	60.71	3,685.70
Total	1207.85		73,265.92
Average	120.79		7,326.59
StDev			85.60

TABLE 5.3   Delta and variance

relates to variability would be to divide the standard deviation by the average, which would give us a ratio of 0.7087, or about 71%, which means that there is a lot of dispersion around that mean. This ratio is called the Coefficient of Variance, or CV, and, while it is a mouthful, the concept is simple: the lower the ratio, the less the dispersion of the data. Remember the example I gave earlier of the party where the average age was 40. A small CV might be 20%, or a standard deviation of 8, while a 71% CV would give me a standard deviation of 28. We will see how this impacts dispersion shortly.

One of the benefits of a normal distribution is that we can estimate the number of data points that fall within a certain range by using these standard deviations. Take a look at this image of a normal distribution:

Each of the vertical lines represents a standard deviation. The μ symbol is the mean, so you can see the first vertical line to the right and the left of the mean is plus or minus one standard deviation, respectively. The second lines represent plus or minus two standard deviations and the third lines represent plus and minus three standard deviations. In a true normal (or near-normal) distribution, we know that approximately 65% of all the data points fall within plus and minus one standard deviation. We also know that approximately 95% fall within plus and minus two standard deviations, and 99.5% fall within three standard deviations.

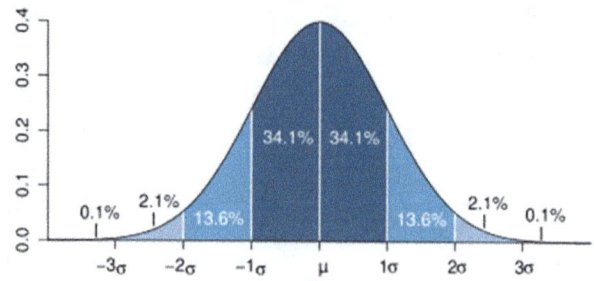

FIGURE 5.6 Normal distribution

Let's go back to our party. With a standard deviation of 8, I could expect that around 65% of everyone at the party was between 32 and 48. Two standard deviations would give me a value of 16, so this would mean that around 95% of the people at the party were between the ages of 24 and 56. And if I stretched this out to three standard deviations (24), I could expect that 99.5% of the party goers would be between the ages of 40 +/- 24, or between 16 and 64. Taking this concept one step further, if I wanted to be able to calculate at what age we could call it an outlier, it would be in the 0.25% tails of this distribution, or greater (and less) than plus and minus 3 standard deviations. So, the low outliers would begin at less than 16 and the high outliers would begin at greater than 64, and what I could expect is that fewer than 0.5% of folks would fall into this category. I hope this makes sense.

Once again, we face the issue of the distribution of the data. In a heavily skewed data set, not only is the average a poor measure of central tendency, the standard deviation can be a poor measure of variability or dispersion. In those cases, where we are relying upon the median rather than the mean, variability is measured differently. There is something called the *interquartile range* (IQR), and this is the range of values between the 25th percentile (1st quartile) and the 75th percentile (3rd quartile). What we do know is that 50% of all the data points fall between these two quartiles and is a great way to visualize the variance of the data. If you look at the age example above, you can see that the IQR for this data set is 8. I get this by subtracting the 25th percentile value (23) from the 75th percentile value (31), which means that approximately 50% of the ages fall between 23 and 31 years old. Calculating outliers using the median and percentiles is a bit different, as well. The calculation may sound a bit more complicated but is easily done. You simply multiply the IQR by 1.5 and then subtract from the 25th percentile, to get the low outlier threshold, and add to the 75th percentile to get the high outlier threshold. In our case, it would look something like this:

1.5 x 8 = 12. 12 subtracted from the 25th percentile (23) = 11 and 12 added to the 75th percentile (31) = 43. This means that the low outlier threshold is less than 12 years old (and there weren't any) and the high threshold for outliers would be anyone older than 43.

Distributions

Any discussion of measures of location or central tendency must begin with a discussion of distributions. A distribution is a visualization of what the data look like when plotted on a graph. For example, do the data tend to accumulate on the left side of the graph or on the right side of the graph? Or are the data equally distributed so that each value represents an equal amount of times is another value? Order the data tend to follow what we often refer to as the bell curve, also called the normal distribution. This is quite important and quite simple to determine by using one of many statistical packages or Microsoft Excel®. Just as a side note, before I get into discussions of Microsoft Excel, I would tell you that if you want to become an expert in data modeling using Excel should read Nate Moore's books (*Better Data, Better Decisions* and *Even Better Data, Better Decisions*) or visit his website: mooresolutionsinc.com. He is, by far, the most knowledgeable person with whom I have worked when it comes to analytics and business intelligence using Excel.

A frequency distribution shows the number of observations falling into each of several ranges or values. These can be portrayed as frequency tables or histograms or other types of graphical representation. Here is an example of what a normal distribution would look like:

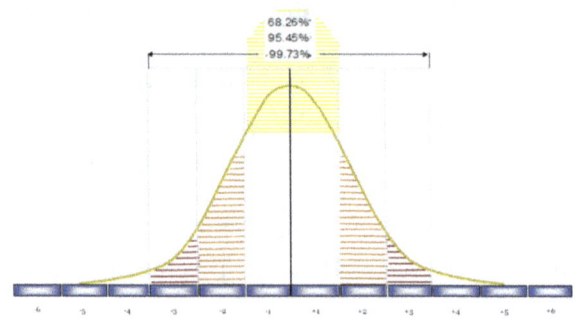

FIGURE 5.7 Normal distribution

Normal distributions have some very convenient characteristics that make them preferable when it comes to data analytics. For example:

1. It is bell-shaped.
2. The mean, median, and mode are equal and located in the center of the distribution.
3. It is unimodal (has only one mode).
4. The curve is symmetric about the mean.
5. The curve is continuous (for each value of x there is a corresponding value of y).
6. The curve never touches the x-axis (goes to infinity).
7. The total area under the curve is 1.00.
8. The area under the curve at 1, 2, and 3 STD is equivalent to 68%, 95% and 99.7% respectively.

Unfortunately, in healthcare, normal distributions are not that, well, normal. We usually see data distributions that are right skewed: the data accumulates to the left with the long right tail like this.

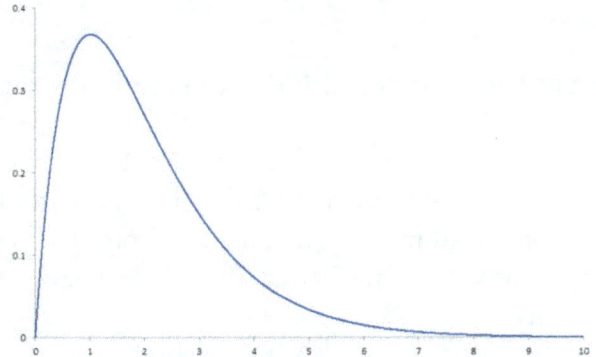

FIGURE 5.8 Long tail, right-skewed data distribution

This occurs in healthcare a lot when looking at things like RVUs, charges, collections, or even patient visits. The reason is that the data are bounded on the left by zero. Think about it; the least amount a physician can get paid for service or procedure is zero dollars. The smallest number of patients that a provider can see in a day is zero. And so, it follows that the smallest number of RVUs that a provider can report in a given period is zero as well. Because of that, the data tend to accumulate more toward the zero side or the left side of the graph than they do the right. And then we have that longer right tail, because while the minimum paid amount may be zero, the maximum could be significantly higher. In these cases, the average is not the most robust or accurate measurement of central tendency. But we will discuss that more later.

We can also see a left skewed, or what's referred to as negative skewed data.

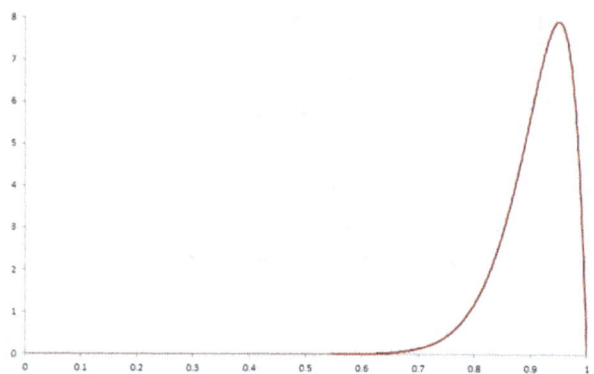

FIGURE 5.9 Long tail, left-skewed data distribution

In a left skewed data, the data points tend to accumulate more toward the right side than the left. I have seen these types of distributions represented by overpaid amounts from chart audits. This is particularly true with a high error rate where there are few zero overpaid amounts.

Here is an example of the difference between a normal distribution and a distribution of data from a real practice. On the left is a distribution that I created using a computer simulation program. I just told it to create a set of values that would define a normal distribution, something you will likely never see in healthcare. On the right is a distribution of frequency data from one of my client's practices. The Y axis reports the magnitude of the frequency: the number of times a certain procedure was reported during the period. The X axis represents each of the procedures reported by the practice.

Now there are many of other types of distributions, but for the purposes of our discussion here, these three should suffice. What we want to know is whether the data are normally distributed or not, but first a discussion on central tendencies and variability.

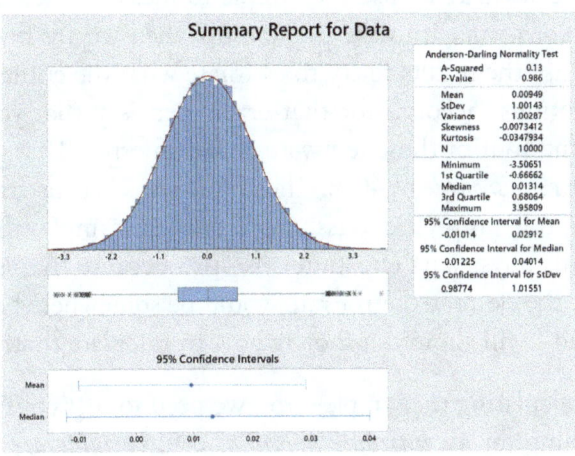

FIGURE 5.10   Summary Report for Data;

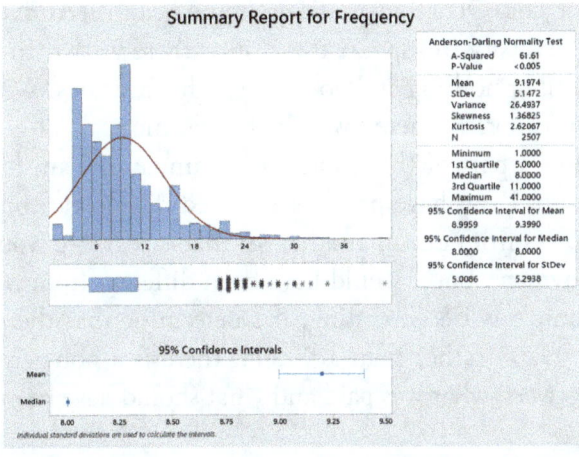

FIGURE 5.11   Summary Report for Frequency

Error and Confidence Interval

Often the data we obtain will be samples of some larger universe. This is very common in healthcare analytics. We do this for audits that involve extrapolation. We sample physician records to estimate productivity. We sample compensation levels and work RVUs and so many other variables. The most important thing to remember when sampling is that there is always going to be *sampling error*. Except in the rarest of cases, the sample is never identical to the population from which it was drawn. If we use the sample to measure the results of that sample and don't infer it to the population, then we are fine. But if we are going to use the results to try to estimate what the entire population looks like we must account for that error. Let's say that you audit ten encounters and four of those ten were coded in error. That gives you an error rate *for that sample* of 40%. The emphasis is because this is for the sample only. You simply can't assume, from this sample, that the error rate for all this physician's encounters is 40% because that is simply not true. In fact, the estimated error rate would be somewhere between 12% and 74%, and I will show you shortly how to calculate that.

When calculating the sample error, we need to first consider whether we are sampling for an *attribute appraisal* or a *variable appraisal*. In an attribute appraisal, we measure each event as a pass/fail. There is no gray area. This might happen if we are auditing for modifier 25; either it was appropriate or not. Or we are auditing home health records; either there was medical necessity to support the visit or there wasn't. In an attribute appraisal, it's all or nothing and no parts can be measures. With a variable appraisal, it is different. Here, we may have some scale of error that can be measured as a part of the whole. For example, if I am looking at an inpatient record, I can have poorly sequenced diagnostic codes that may change the DRG from one to another. In that case, there would still have been some payment, but it would have been different from zero. Another common example is E&M coding; if I determine that the code should have been a 99203 rather than a 99204, there is a non-zero impact, or difference, between what was paid and what should have been paid.

There are some basic margin-of-error rules that go like this:

- The larger the sample, the smaller the error.
- The smaller the variance, the smaller the error.

This becomes clearer when you look at the formula for each. Let's start with the formula for an attribute appraisal:

$$SE = \sqrt{\frac{p(1-p)}{n}}$$

Figure 5.12 Formula for an attribute appraisal

SE stands for the sample error. The *p* is the probability or rate that event occurs and (1-*p*) is just that: the probability the event occurs subtracted from one. Remember, *p* must be between 0 and 1. This means that the probability is always somewhere between 0% and 100%. The *n* represents the number of data points used in the sample. Let's take an example and see how it plays out.

In a chart review, a practice finds out that six out of thirty encounters did not meet medical necessity. As such, each failed the review. This equates to a coding error rate of 20%. Using the formula above, we have:

- $p = 0.2$ (20%)
- $(1-p) = 0.8$ (1 - .2)
- $n = 30$ (the number of encounters reviewed

The sample error = $p(1-p)/n$ = 0.16/30 = .0053. The square root of .0053 is 0.073, or 7.3%. This means that our sample error puts our estimate somewhere between 12.7% (20% - 7.3%) and 27.3%.

The formula for a variable estimate is a bit different. It is:

$$SE_{\bar{x}} = \frac{s_x}{\sqrt{n}}$$

FIGURE 5.13 Formula for a variable estimate

Where SE_x is the sample error of the mean, s_x is the standard deviation of the mean and n is, once again, the number of data points. In this case, rather than getting the square root of the result from the calculation, we only take the square root of the number of data points in the sample. Let's look at an example of this. Let's say that I want to get an estimate of the fee that different physicians are charging for 99213 in some geographic area. I draw a random sample of 50 practices, and I get the standard fee for each one. I then take those 50 fees and get the average and the standard deviation. Let's say the average is $82.40 and the standard deviation is $15.55. For the purpose of this example, we are going to assume a normal distribution, so we know that around 65% of the fees fall between $66.85 and $97.95. This is one standard deviation plus and minus the mean. But that does not measure error, only dispersion. Following the formula above, I divide the standard deviation ($15.55) by the square root of the number of data points on the sample (30). It looks like $15.55/7.07 = 2.20. So, my sample error is between $$80.20 and $84.60. I could also divide it by the mean and estimate my error rate at 2.67%.

Now, I hope you can see why we use the two rules mentioned above. To reduce the sample error, I need to either increase the sample size or decrease the variability. The latter is about impossible to do on a random sample because the variability in the universe (or the population) is what it is. I can't do much to affect that. But I can increase my sample size. If I doubled to 100 data points, the SE would be 15.55 / 10, or 1.5 rather than 2.2 because now I would be dividing by 10 (the square root of 100) instead of 7.07 (the square root of 50).

The final idea around variability that I want to discuss is something called the *z-score*. This is a measure of standard distance in a normally distributed database. I am sure that many of us have seen data represented with *confidence intervals*, whether studies or biostatistical research or even the CERT study, which I will discuss shortly. The most common confidence intervals we encounter for our work are 80%, 90%, 95%, and 99%. For example, in an extrapolation audit, such as we would experience with a ZPIC, UPIC or RAC, the overpayment is normally calculated based on a 90% confidence interval, which may be of benefit to the provider if, in fact, the sample is proper, and the calculations are accurate. So, the confidence interval (note the word *interval*) measures a range of values surrounding the central point estimate: in this case, the mean. Maybe I am trying to estimate the number of work RVUs I expect to report next year for all my providers, or even for a single provider. From my sample, rather than report an exact point estimate, I use a range, maybe a low of 4,890 to a high of 5,650, both of which surround a mean value of 5,270. Many people will exemplify the confidence interval by saying something like, "I am 90% confident that my estimate is correct." I believe that this usage is a misleading, and even incorrect, representation of what the data really means. More appropriate would be to state that: "If I were to repeat this same study 100 times, my point estimate would be between the low and high range 95% of the time." (This assumes we are talking about a 95% confidence interval.) This range is referred to as the *margin of error*.

Let's look at a few real examples. A good place to start is with the CERT study. CERT stands for Comprehensive Error Rate Testing and is a study conducted annually by CMS to estimate the amount of money that is being paid out improperly. The way they do this is to randomly select some number of claims for all providers and provider types (e.g. physicians, SNFs, acute care hospitals, DME, etc.) and then, for each claim, request the documentation from the provider. An auditor then reviews the claims and, using Medicare guidelines, determines whether the documentation supported the paid amount or whether the claim was paid improperly. Here is the CERT summary report for 2017:

Claim Type	Claims Sampled	Claims Reviewed	Total Payment	Projected Improper Payment	Improper Payment Rate	95% Confidence Interval	Percent of Overall Improper Payments
Part A (Total)	29,756	22,001	$275.6	$22.7	8.2%	7.5% - 9.0%	62.7%
Part A (Excluding Hospital IPPS)	8,626	7,501	$161.3	$18.2	11.3%	10.1% - 12.6%	50.4%
Part A (Hospital IPPS)	21,130	14,500	$114.3	$4.5	3.9%	3.5% - 4.3%	12.3%
Part B	17,550	17,000	$97.0	$9.9	10.2%	9.3% - 11.0%	27.2%
DMEPOS	11,357	11,001	$8.2	$3.7	44.6%	42.5% - 46.7%	10.1%
Overall	58,663	50,002	$380.8	$36.2	9.5%	8.9% - 10.1%	100.0%

TABLE 5.4 CERT summary report for 2017

According to this table, the overall Improper Payment Rate (or error rate) was 9.5%. This means that of the $380.8 million dollars associated to those 50,000 claims that were reviewed, some $36 million (9.5%) should not have been paid. Notice the next column, the one with the heading "95% Confidence Interval." The range is 8.9% to 10.1%. This means that if CMS were to pull 100 more random samples of 50,002 from the same population and calculated a confidence interval for each, we could expect the *point estimate* to be between the population estimates in 95 out of 100 samples. This means that in only 5%, or in 1 out of 20 samples, would the point estimate be either higher or lower due to something other than just normal variability. Another way we could state this would be to say that we are 95% confident that the actual point estimate for the entire population is between 8.9% and 10.1%.

Why is this important to us? Let's use physicians as an example and look at the table above for part B. Here, it shows the point estimate for the error rate at 10.2% with the 95% confidence interval of 9.3% to 11%. Let's say your practice gets audited and the auditor comes up with an error rate of 35% or 45%. Remember, since this is a randomized national study, which included your data in the population and could have been selected as part of the sample, we would expect that these results would apply to you as well as any other practice. Remember what the confidence interval means. In this case, to simplify things just a bit, we could say that if the auditor were to pull at random the same number of claims from our population 100 times and conducted 100 audits, in 95 out of those 100, the error rate should have been somewhere between 9.3% and 11%. This means that we are either one of the unlucky one out of twenty that had an error rate that much higher than the other 95, or the auditors did not conduct their audit in good faith. I would opine that the latter is usually the case, since we see a reversal rate in favor of the provider of well over 50%. The reason I mention this is because if your organization is audited, particularly when an extrapolation is involved, these types of errors at the sample level can result in millions of dollars of improper overpayment demands at the population level.

Hopefully, you can see that the purpose of the confidence interval is to validate some point estimate; it tells us how far off our estimate is likely to be within difference samples. The width of the interval gives us some idea as to how uncertain we are about that estimate. In general, the higher the confidence interval, the wider the range, which makes logical sense, because if I give myself more latitude, I can be more confident in the results. Let's look at an example. Southwest Airlines operates over five hundred Boeing 737-300 airplanes. What I want is for you to guess the wingspan on that plane (don't search Google for it!), and then tell me how confident you are that you are right. I couldn't give you a point estimate and have any confidence that I was right, but I could give you a range in feet and assign a level of confidence to that range. For example, I am 99% confident that the wingspan is somewhere between 50 feet and a football field (300 feet). Seems a bit of a crazy range, but hey, look how confident I am that the real number is somewhere in that range. Maybe I am 95% confident that it is somewhere between 75 feet and 150 feet. Or 80% confident that it is between 90 feet and 120 feet. See, the narrower the range, the less confident I become, and this is also true with how confidence intervals work in mathematics. The lower bound of the 90% confidence interval is closer to the mean than the lower bound of a 95% or 99% confidence interval. To narrow the confidence interval, you can decrease your variability, as discussed above, or you can increase the sample size.

In physician compensation models, using the confidence interval is especially important. Let's say that you are developing a compensation plan based on work RVUs. For your general surgeons, you expect them to produce 4,852 work RVUs per year to be considered as a full-time employee. You decide that if they report more than the 4,852, they qualify for a bonus, but if they report less than 4,852, they get dinged. Just think about how unrealistic (and unfair) this is to both the practice and the doc. Normal variability alone will account for higher and lower work RVU values, and so a physician gets rewarded or penalized if the target moves by one or two work RVUs, and this will *always* happen and will be due to something outside of their control. If we use confidence intervals, however, we can solve that problem.

Let's say for this example, the lower bound of the 95% confidence interval is 4,435 and the upper bound is 5,124. Now, what we are saying is that, if the provider reports work RVUs between the lower and the upper value, they are considered as a 1 FTE employee. The bonus kicks in when they report more than 5,124 work RVUs, and they get dinged when they report fewer than 4,435 work RVUs. This is looking at when they are statistically significantly higher or lower than the mean. That range in between is part of the sampling error we discussed above and will always exist when we do sampling. And since this is due to normal variation, we don't want to reward or punish a provider for things that are outside of their control. I call this the "nod is as good as a wink to a blind horse" method.

Let's look at it from an auditing perspective. Let's say a practice gets audited by a ZPIC and of the 30 charts they audited, they found an overpayment amount that calculated to $104.32 per claim. That's the average. Let's say that they drew the sample from a universe of 10,000 claims. If you were to take the average and multiplied by those 10,000 claims, you would get an extrapolated overpayment estimate of $1,043,200. Now, let's say that the lower bound was $84.60. Multiply this number by the 10,000 claims, and you get an estimated overpayment amount of $840,600. This is a reduction in overpayment demand of over $202,000. That makes a substantial difference.

Precision

The final topic I wanted to talk about is precision. *Precision* refers to how close estimates from different samples are to each other. It also estimates how repeatable those results would be from sample to sample. What we want to know is how precise is that estimate of central tendency. In our audit, we want to know how precise the estimate of $104.32 per claim is. If the precision is really poor, meaning that it's not very repeatable and it's not very accurate, it could mean that the entire extrapolation would be worthless. Think about it, even if we calculated a lower bound of some confidence interval, if the data were some variable that we didn't have a reliable point estimate for the average of, then we wouldn't have a very reliable lower bound for the confidence interval. Even though the auditor might say that using the lower bound benefits the practice, if the data don't exhibit any degree of homogeneity, then the extrapolation should be disregarded in its entirety.

One way to measure precision is simply to take the difference between the average (or the mean) and the lower bound of the confidence interval, and then divide that back by the average. In this case, we would subtract the $84.60 from $104.32 to get $19.72. Divide this by $104.32, and we get a precision of 18.9%. Is this a good number or a bad number? In precision, the smaller the percentage the better. A small percentage means we're more accurate, while a large percentage means we're less accurate. Corporate integrity agreements that are in force by the Office of Inspector General say that the precision cannot exceed 25%. In most of the audits in which I have been a statistical expert, the auditors have a target of 10%. According to the Government Accounting Office, and even CMS, published in the Federal Register in 2008, the target precision is 2.5%. Remember, a really large precision percent means that the data are highly variable and likely should not be used for extrapolation. The key point is to keep this in mind as you work through your analytics and to question the viability and repeatability of the results you get from data sets that exhibit poor precision.

Chapter 6
Predicting like a Pro

Predicting is both an art and a science and covers the gamut from the Oracle of Delphi, astrology, tarot cards, and Ouija Boards, to the advanced statistical sciences of predictive analytics, artificial intelligence, and machine learning. Remember the Danish aphorism mentioned previously, "It is hard to predict, especially the future." The truth of that statement holds true for all generations. Predicting *is* hard and predicting the future is the hardest of all, yet we spend an enormous amount of time focused on doing just that.

In chaos theory, there is this point, beyond which predicting becomes nearly impossible. This is the *prediction horizon*, which define how far ahead the model can predict the future. While the topic can get quite dense quite fast, the basic idea has to do with how well we are able to control our environment, and how well we are able to adapt to change, both expected and unexpected. In meteorology, for example, we inherently know (and it bears out in the proof) that the further we go out into the future, the more difficult it is to predict the weather, or at least predict with any degree of accuracy. Weather is a complex system and there are many interrelationships that can alter the prediction at most any time. But the closer we get to the predictive moment, the more accurate our prediction becomes, and that is because of our ability to adjust our model to those changes.

Around the middle of September 2017, Hurricane Irma made landfall on Marco Island, Florida. I live a bit north of Tampa, and we had been preparing, on and off, for nearly a week. I say, "on and off," because it was not clear, at least that far out, where Irma was going and where it would make landfall. At 10 days out, the spaghetti models looked like this:

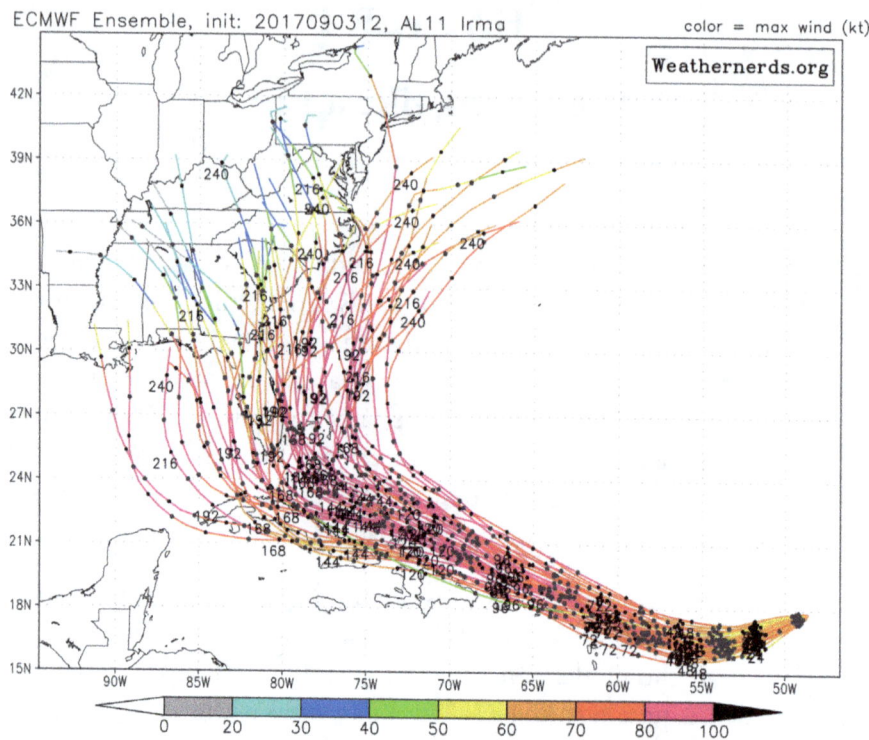

FIGURE 6.1 Hurricane Irma predicted paths 10 days out from Florida landfall, weathernerds.org

At that point, it was uncertain as to whether Irma would make landfall at all, much less in Florida. At about five days out, the models shifted the track of the storm more easterly and so the east coast of Florida moved more aggressively to prepare for the storm.

Predicting like a Pro

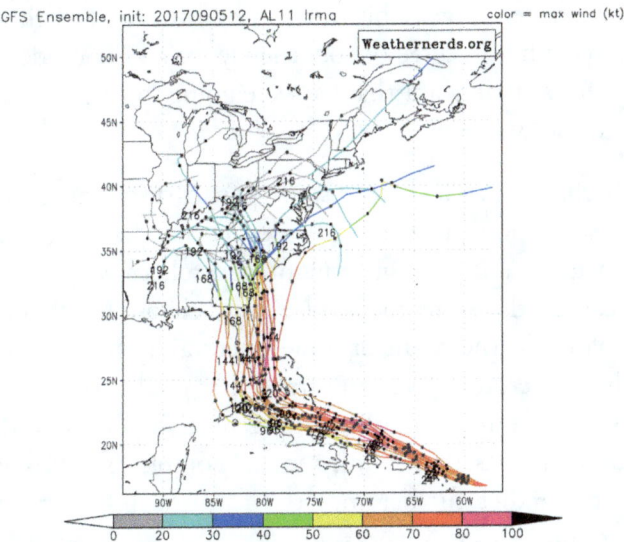

Figure 6.2   Hurricane Irma predicted paths 5 days out from Florida landfall, weathernerds.org

Then, at only three days out, the models shifted west, as shown below:

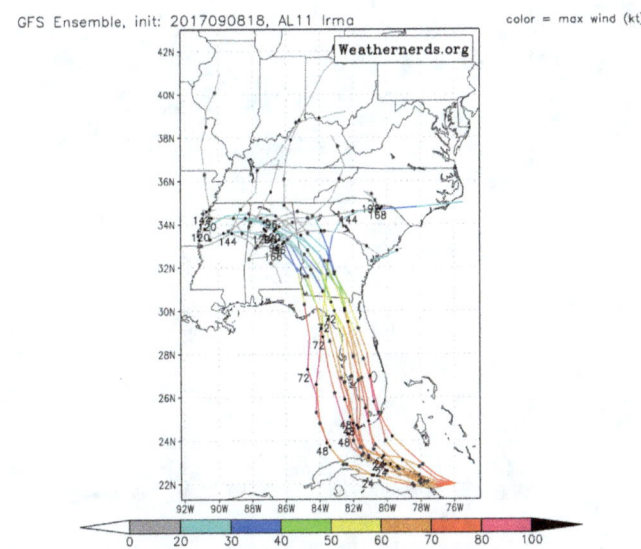

Figure 6.3   Hurricane Irma predicted paths 3 days out from Florida landfall, weathernerds.org

Now we started to get a bit worried, and the final track, only a day before, showed a high degree of congruency for all the models. We were quite confident at that point that we were going to be in the path of the storm . . . and we were!

In this chaos model, there is some perturbation, or disturbance to the state at some point in time. If we don't dampen that perturbation, it begins to grow and can get out of control, causing the model to fail. This causes the state to devolve into chaos. Much of the time, this perturbation is the result of some uncertainty in our model, so by reducing that uncertainty, we can extend that prediction horizon, which is a great benefit from a management perspective. The goal, then, is not to eliminate chaos, as that is inherent in complex systems, but rather to be able to predict further into the future. The illustration below demonstrates how this this works.

Remediation comes from something known as Ashby's Law of Requisite Variety. The concept deals with readiness and planning. It is

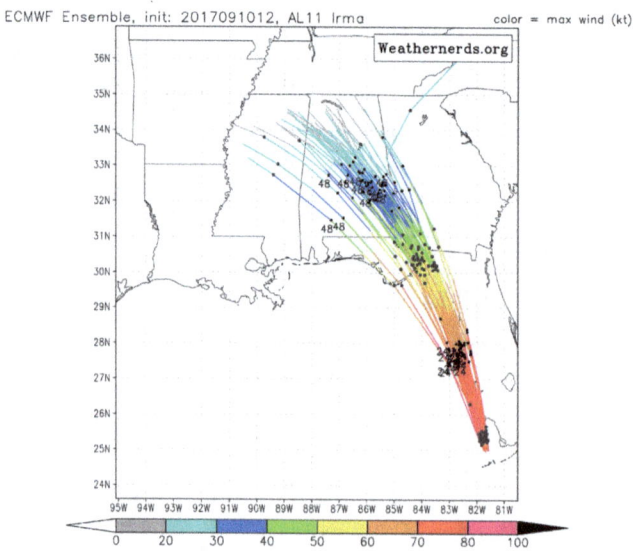

FIGURE 6.4   Hurricane Irma predicted paths 1 day out from Florida landfall, weathernerds.org

about our toolbox and having the tools necessary to be able to tamp down that perturbation when it occurs. The toolbox grows over time, with experience, and the better we get at managing these tools, the better we become at making good predictions.

A great example of this deals with why grandparents have a better time with their grandkids than they did with their kids. And as a grandfather, I can attest to this. Most young adults can manage four basic disruptions that occur with an infant. They are hungry, they are tired, they are soiled, or they are sick. And it doesn't take long before an attentive parent learns the difference in the baby's cries, which identifies which of these disturbances (or perturbations) are occurring. If the baby is hungry, the parent feeds them. If the baby is tired, the baby gets put to bed. If the baby soils its diaper, the parent changes it; and if the baby is sick, the parent takes them to the doctor. Those are for inherently functional tools within their toolbox. But what happens when that little infant begins to grow? I can tell you from my experience raising four daughters. Perturbations appear that I never expected, and more importantly, that I didn't know how to handle. I didn't have the requisite tools to be able to deal with the disruption in the state, such as relationships, and as a result my home moved into chaos. Now I have grandchildren. I have a very full toolbox, and so, when disruptions occur with the grandchildren, I put on my "been there, done that" T-shirt and rarely do things move to chaos.

From a management perspective, it's the same idea. Some disruption occurs in the state; maybe an audit or a technology problem or personnel issues or billing and coding issues. Experienced managers who have dealt with these issues in the past have the requisite variety of tools to be able to tamp down these perturbations and prevent the state from going to chaos. This experience helps to reduce the uncertainty around the decisions that we make, even about the future, ensuring that, more times than not, the outcome is positive.

This chapter is not about predictive analytics *per se*, which deals with advanced statistical methods. It is about predicting using the tools

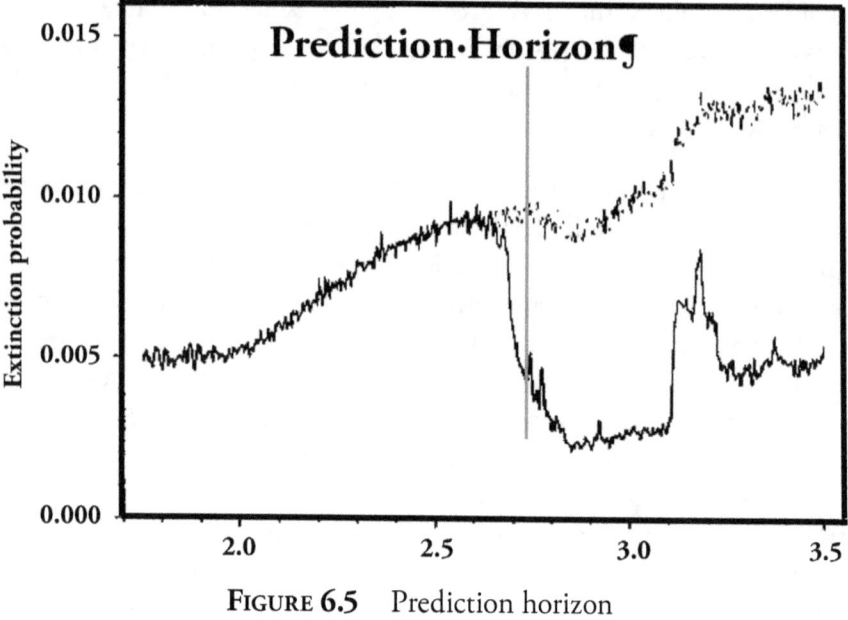

FIGURE 6.5 Prediction horizon

that we have in hand. There are lots of methods available to us, some mathematical and some not, that allow us to become better at predicting future outcomes. These include:

- Linear decomposition
- Scanning method
- Prediction by analogy
- Extrapolation method
- Trend analysis
- Time-series analysis
- Scenario method
- The Fermi Method
- Delphi survey method
- Diversity Prediction Theorem

Linear Decomposition

Linear decomposition relies upon the ability to deconstruct (or decompose) an aggregate whole into its component parts. The idea is that the value of the parts together equal or approximate the value of the whole. For example, if I measured the length of your knee to the bottom of your foot, and your knee to your hipbone, and your hipbone to your shoulder, and then your shoulder to your head, and I added all these measurements together, it would likely give me a pretty accurate indication of your total height. For this to work, we have to be able to either measure or estimate whatever the value is for each of the parts.

For example, predicting what it will cost to open a new medical practice works well with linear decomposition. I might take the lease or purchase value of the property, the cost of the equipment necessary to run the practice, the salaries and benefits for the different staff involved, an estimate of the variable expenses tied up in things like supplies and reagents, and then maybe the technology required in the form of a practice management system or an EHR. Adding each of these parts up, assuming I've included all that there are, I should arrive at a reasonable estimate of the cost of setting up and running a medical practice.

Another example may involve trying to estimate the productivity loss you can expect when implementing a new EHR. We might, for example, look at the training time required for the staff members. If your billing and coding people are involved, estimating productivity loss at that level is relatively linear. Same goes with physicians. The time that physicians spend in training is time that they are not seeing patients, and it's not that difficult to calculate revenue per unit of service and apply that toward the lost time. You can also look at the number of providers that might be involved and estimate some productivity loss resulting from bringing the EHR up to speed. When you add all these components together, you should be able to get a reasonable estimate as to what the cost of the productivity loss will be.

On the positive side, we often know all the parts that make up a whole. And there are lots of resources available to us to research those parts values. We can use search engines to look at prior studies, read white papers, talk to vendors, and even speak with managers of other practices that are engaged in the same types of change models we are looking at. As long as the model is linear, meaning that there is a one-to-one relationship between the value and the parts, we are actually quite good at accurately predicting the composite value.

On the downside, sometimes it's difficult to know the value of each of the parts. On our EHR example, it's not always easy to predict what productivity loss might be at the physician level because it involves physician behavior and their willingness to adapt to a new technology. On the example of opening a new practice, we may have uncertainties around the lease price per square foot based upon what the market is doing at the time. We also might find out that the value of the parts does not always equal the value of the whole. This is often the case in nonlinear decomposition problems. Which brings us to the consideration that not all the interactions will be linear, and we need to be able to recognize when that is the case.

Prediction by Analogy

When we try *prediction by analogy*, what we are doing is estimating the value of a given entity based on similar values in a different entity. If I was trying to estimate what the miles per gallon might be on a particular vehicle, I could look at other vehicles that had similar size engine and a similar weight and use that as a starting point. Often, I have run into this when people are trying to estimate the RVU value for a procedure that does not have an official RVU value. What you can do is look at other procedures that are similar and then adjust the RVU value for those procedures based on how much more consumptive or less consumptive this procedure might be.

The same holds true when retrying to estimate how long it will take to perform a new procedure. Or even how long it might take to see a new patient with a particular diagnosis. We can look at the time it takes for similar procedures to be performed and how long it takes to see new patients with similar diagnoses.

We can even use the example from before about how much it might cost to open a new medical practice by looking at the cost that others have incurred opening their medical practices. If those practices were larger, then we can downsize our estimate, and if they were smaller, then we can upsize our estimate. The thing to remember is that whenever were trying to predict, the further we go out in time, the greater the uncertainty is going to be. In prediction by analogy, the less analogous the other entity, the greater the uncertainty around our estimates.

In prediction by analogy, it's always good to get more people involved, because different people see relationships differently. They live in different boxes, and so it gives you a broader perspective. And even if we can't estimate precisely the central tendencies, analogous measurements are quite effective at setting upper and lower boundaries. Even though I might not be able to predict what the cost might be for some event, I could more accurately determine what the minimum cost might be as well as the maximum cost. Or in the example of assigning an RVU to a code that doesn't have one, what would be the minimum RVU value versus the maximum RVU value?

The other point is that known information is known. Meaning that it can be verified, so at least we know we're dealing with facts versus anecdote. There are also some problems with this method. For example, it only focuses on the similarities and not the differences. The differences can sway our estimates quite a bit, so we have to take that into consideration. Another problem has to do with the confirmation bias, where we try to fit an event into an analogy even when it doesn't fit. The biggest problem with this method happens when we accept assumptions without testing or validating them.

Extrapolation Method

Pretty much anyone who has been subjected to a coding and billing audit knows about extrapolation. Extrapolation is an estimation of the value based on extending unknown sequence of values or facts be on the area that is certainly known. For example, an auditor may come in and pull 30 claims at random from a universe of 10,000 claims. They analyze those 30 claims and come up with an average overpayment based on coding errors of $100 per claim. Extrapolation would occur when they took that known sequence from the sample—that $100 per claim—and multiplied it by the 10,000 claims in the universe. Now the demand is $1 million, but only a fraction of the claims that account for that million dollars have been audited. Extrapolation is more estimation than it is prediction.

To convert extrapolation to prediction, we would want to know what the estimated overpayment would be for the next 10,000 claims not coded or billed yet. The reason we don't do this is because of the huge amount of uncertainty surrounding that type of a prediction. The upper and lower bounds would be so wide as to render the extrapolation useless. So, for extrapolation to be successful we must know that the sequence or the sample is representative of the universe to which that prediction or estimation will fall. I've seen this used a lot when trying to predict the amount of time and effort expended by physicians within an organization by taking a sample of work RVUs and extrapolating it to all the physicians within the organization. I also see this done in internal audits.

For example, an organization may audit some number of claims or beneficiaries and come up with an error rate. Then they try to extrapolate or expand that error rate to the entire organization. One of the salient benefits of extrapolation is that it's based on scientific principles, and therefore it's replicable. So, when the government comes in and does an extrapolation audit, as a statistician, I should be able to replicate their findings. Also, the accuracy of an extrapolation is known and is calculated using standard statistical methods.

When it comes to case law, both the statistical community and the courts accept the validity of extrapolation. Sampling methodology is the biggest problem with extrapolation. To begin with, sampling is that it cannot be entirely precise, and it always has some probability of missing critical elements. In fact, since sampling itself has so many potential pitfalls, it is the number one impediment to accurate extrapolation. If you are going to engage in this method, you should have—or you should engage someone that does have—a good understanding of sampling methodology.

Trend Analysis

Trending is one of my favorite methods, and this is the process of comparing data over time to identify results or trends, which are then used to predict events and values beyond the end of the sequence. This is one of the big differences between this method and extrapolation. We see this a lot in budgeting. When a manager or department head is trying to predict what their expenses will be next year, they often will do a trend analysis rather than just take some average of what was spent the year prior. Trending allows us to see whether patterns are moving up or moving down; for example, whether costs are increasing or decreasing over time. If I'm working on a physician compensation model that includes work RVUs, I might want to be able to estimate how many work RVUs will be reported next year. This is important when trying to establish a compensation pool and particularly to calculate bonus amounts per work RVU.

In this case, I would look at the trend of work RVUs over the year, and then use that to continue that trend moving forward. I might also want to know how long it will take a new physician to cover their expenses. One way to do this is by looking at trends from other physicians or to simply track and trend this physician's revenue versus costs, and then predict how much longer in the future it will take. This is also known as *time series analysis* and there are many software programs, including Microsoft Excel, that allow you to do this and to include uncertainty around your projections. In fact, it is important to remember that in all these estimation methods, we are predicting a range of events rather than an exact point estimate.

On the plus side, this is a popular and widespread method, hence the many software solutions available. It's also based on historical data, which can be validated and verified. Any future predictions have got to be dependent upon reliable prior data that allows us to verify that the trends. Because we are once again creating a range of estimates, we are allowing for error, so we don't *overfit* the model. On the negative side, and we all know this is true because we have experienced it many times, no matter how accurate the historical data are, they are not always indicative of future events. Part of this problem involves the difficulty in predicting turning points or seminal events in a timeseries data set. It may also require the ability to do seasonal adjustments if those impact the values. And because of the inherent nature of perturbations and chaos, there is a predictive horizon that is not always known *a priori*.

Scenario Method

I have already given an example of the scenario method when I was sharing the decision-making process when considering purchasing an EHR, and the impacts of whether a practice would remain small, merge with a larger system, or close. These were the three possible scenarios the physicians imagined. The *scenario method* is about visualizing what future conditions or events are probable, as well as what their consequences or effects would be like, and how to respond and/or benefit from them. One of the conditions of the scenario method is that it must be physically, socially, and politically plausible. I won't rehash the same examples that I gave before but remember that it was about what type of EHR system would fit into the practice based on those three scenarios that were given.

I think a good application for this would be to imagine what the impact would be they replaced CPT codes with ICD-##-PCS codes. It would be a complete paradigm shift to accommodate the structure and organization of the PCS codes. For example, what would be the time and cost involved in retraining? How about all the certifications held that would no longer be valid? Or what about, from a vendor perspective, having to retool all the software to work in a completely new and completely different structure for coding outpatient services? The question we are asking is this: given what we understand about the present, what is going on now, what would we expect to happen if one of these different events were to occur or a different trend were to develop?

The biggest advantage with the scenario method is that it doesn't necessarily tell you what you should or should not do. It just gives you some idea of what may or may not happen. This opens the door for more exploration and doesn't bind you to a solution. You can also have many different potential outcomes and events. There can be an infinite number of future possibilities. When the stakes are high, and there is a high uncertainty, the scenario method is especially useful.

One of the problems that I have with this method is that the predictions can be extremely broad in chronological, geographical, and thematic scope. And because this is a nonlinear approach, the problems of complexity can obfuscate what would otherwise be obvious observations. Also, uncertainty and impact can be highly subjective, so the question is: who chooses those futures? In this scenario method, it's always good to have a diverse group of people providing their ideas and their input. Remember, unlike trend analysis or extrapolation, which can be defined by mathematical models, the scenario method is open to individual vision and interpretation.

The Fermi Method (Dimensional Analysis)

Now we come upon my very favorite method for prediction without the use of advanced statistical methods. A Fermi problem is a multistep problem that can be solved in a variety of ways, and whose solution requires the estimation of key pieces of information. Named after Enrico Fermi, a Nobel prize-winning physicist, who, in addition to the contributions that he made to science, was also known for his uncanny ability to make good predictions or approximations with little or no real data. This is a great method for solving problems that most people have never really considered.

There is one well-known company that I know of that will ask questions as part of their preemployment interviews to see how well a person is able to solve an otherwise nonlinear problem. For example, how many golf balls would fit into a school bus? It seems like a pretty strange question and not a problem that anyone would ever really have to solve. But let's try it anyway.

Don't Do Something, Just Stand There

We know that there are different sized school buses, but let's estimate what the interior dimensions are for the school bus that you remember riding on. I know that the width is larger than the distance between my fingertips when I stretch my arms out, and in fact, I know that it was about a quarter of that wider. So, I'm going to estimate that the width of the bus is about 7 ½ feet, or 90 inches. My best guess is that each window is about 2.5 feet in length. I estimate there are 10 windows on the bus, which gives an interior length of 25 feet. If I multiply the length times the width, I get about 187.5 ft.^{2}.

The next thing to do is estimate the height of the bus. I know I can stand up in the bus, so I know it's taller than 6 feet, but not much more than that. I'm going to guess 6 feet 6 inches. So, I multiply the 187.5 ft^2 times the 6.5 feet, and I get a volume of about 1,219 ft^3. I know that there is 1,728 in^3 in a cubic foot, so doing the math, I come up with 2,106,432 in^3 for the interior of the bus.

Then I have to do is to figure out how much room those seats take up. I am going to estimate about 10%, which brings my area estimate to 1,685,146 in^3. The next step is to calculate the area of a golf ball. I don't golf, but I did measure the radius of a golf ball at about 0.85 inches. This would give me an area of 2.5 in^3 by using the formula of 4/3 times pi times the radius. You can also cheat by looking all the values up on a search engine, but that takes away a lot of the fun!

We now have enough information to approximate the number of golf balls that would fit on our school bus. We take the area of the bus (1,685,146), divided by the area of the golf ball (2.5), and we get an answer of 674,058 golf balls. But let's go one step further. A golf ball is round, and so when you stack them together, there's going to be this space in between that is filled with air. I may be wrong, but I'm going to guess that accounts for about 20% of the volume in the bus, which would give me a final answer of 539,247 golf balls. Am I right? Most likely, no. But I'm a lot closer now than I was when asked the question.

The most famous Fermi problem is calculating how many piano tuners there are in Chicago. I love doing this live, because when you ask that question all you see are blank stares. First, how relevant could this question possibly be? And who in the world has ever even thought about it? That's what makes it such a great test of this method. But since I've seen this problem worked through so many times, I'm going to put a little bit of a twist to it, and instead ask how many piano tuners are there in Los Angeles? Let's apply the same dimensional analysis that we did with the golf balls. (This requires you to look some of this up on the internet.)

My best estimate was 3.2 million households in the greater Los Angeles area. According to the research I looked at, about 20% of those households will have a piano, which is 640,000. I discover that 10% will tune their pianos on average once a year, which brings us to 64,000 piano tunings every year. My research shows that it takes about two hours to tune an average piano, so that's about 128,000 hours. If you figure a typical work year is 2,080 hours, that comes out to 61 work years. Which means that there would need to be about 61 piano tuners in the greater Los Angeles area. Once again, am I right? Most likely I'm not. But I'm a lot less uncertain than I was when first addressing the question.

Well, that's enough fun for me. In our industry, we might use this to estimate physicians needed in a given community or estimate the number of people that will visit emergency rooms this year. What I like most about this method is that, most often, it is a quick and simple initial method to use before embarking on some formal approach. It also helps us to identify in advance where errors may be located within these types of complex calculations. And normally, the tools and the information we need are readily available.

Think about it, in the prior two examples, we could've looked all this up on the internet and all we would've needed was a calculator. But we also must keep in mind that most often these answers may not be overly accurate. For example, if there are 75 piano tuners in the Los Angeles area, then that means I might have been off by 20%. We must determine how important accuracy is. We also have to make a lot of assumptions, so in both of those examples, if I was wrong in any of the estimates of the parts, it could quickly multiply that small error into a large error. For example, if I was off by even 10% on my estimate of the area of a golf ball, it would've made a difference of tens of thousands in the end. I think the biggest problem I have found with this method is that it is a lazy alternative to what should often be a more rigorous effort.

Diversity Prediction Theorem

This is another one of my favorite methods, albeit a bit more complex and involving a bit more mathematics than the others. The *diversity prediction theorem,* introduced by Professor Scott Page—a social scientist and the Leonid Hurwicz, Collegiate Professor of Complex Systems, Political Science, and Economics at the University of Michigan. Professor Paige is one of my heroes. I have used this method to build certain cohort groups that I use within my risk-based auditing application. In general, the diversity prediction theorem states that a diverse crowd will always be more accurate than a single individual or its average member. Mathematically speaking, it states that the *crowd squared error* equals the *average individual squared error* minus the *diversity of the predictions.* Therefore, it means that when the diversity of a group or team or an organization is large, the error of the crowd is small. The proof is that, given a crowd of predictive models, the collective error will equal the average individual error minus the prediction diversity. I apply this method to my teambuilding courses and engagements.

We can measure the diversity of a team by looking at specific *heuristics* or rules that people use to make decisions and solve problems. Some examples of heuristics are:

- If you are having difficulty solving a problem, reduce it to its smallest components.
- Two heads are better than one.
- Too many cooks spoil the broth.
- Measure twice, cut once.

The greater the *heuristic diversity,* sometimes called the *cognitive diversity,* the better the outcomes. This is specifically true when doing problem-solving, prediction and projection, or preference aggregation.

Predicting like a Pro

Without getting too far into the weeds mathematically, a fitting example of this is trying to guess the number of jellybeans in a jar. I know you have seen this at trade shows or conferences, where the vendors will have jellybeans out in some container, and they'll ask you to guess how many there are, and you win a prize if you're the closest. When I do this live, I have asked people what methods they might use to guess the number of jellybeans in that container. Here are some of the responses;

- Count the number of jellybeans around the circumference of the container and estimate the number in that row and then multiply it by the number of rows of jellybeans.
- Estimate the volume of the container based on its shape and size and divide that by the estimated volume of a jellybean.
- Guess.
- Look it up online.

So, what's the best method? It would be hanging around by the booth and writing down everyone's guesses and then taking the average. Let's say that the actual number was 1,120. Invoking the diversity prediction theorem as a proof, it would look something like this:

Player	Guess	Average Error	Diversity (Ave. Indiv. Error)	Crowd Error	Percent Variance
1	850.00	73,441.00	59,146.24	14,294.76	-24.17%
2	1,265.00	20,736.00	29,515.24	(8,779.24)	12.85%
3	605.00	266,256.00	238,339.24	27,916.76	-46.03%
4	1,390.00	72,361.00	88,090.24	(15,729.24)	24.00%
5	1,510.00	151,321.00	173,722.24	22,401.24	34.70%
6	612.00	259,081.00	231,553.44	27,527.56	-45.41%
7	900.00	48,841.00	37,326.24	11,514.76	-19.71%
8	1,450.00	108,241.00	127,306.24	(19,065.24)	29.35%
9	955.00	27,556.00	19,099.24	8,456.76	-14.81%
10	1,395.00	75,076.00	91,038.24	(16,007.24)	24.44%
Individual		110,291.00	109,518.16	772.84	
Crowd Average		772.84			-2.48%
Crowd Sq. Error				772.84	
Actual					

TABLE 6.1 Diversity prediction theorem table

What we've done is taken each of the individual guesses and calculated the average, which in this case is 1,093.2. Then we calculate the difference between each guess and the average, and we square that number. We do the same thing with the actual value. We then calculate the *average error* and the *diversity*. In this case, you can see that the *crowd square error* is less than the *squared error for the individuals*. And the way we do this is to take the *average error* minus the *diversity* and that equals the *crowds' error*.

This is a great method to use within teams or other types of diverse organizations. It relies upon the cognitive diversity of the members and therefore it is imperative that diversity is given precedence over skills or knowledge. Pretty much anyone can be trained to do a job and to do it correctly, but if you get too many people who think the same way and solve problems the same way, limiting that diversity, you will never achieve the level of success that you would with a more diverse crowd.

I would direct you back to the beginning of this book and have you ask yourself a question: are you a fox or a hedgehog? And is the team you're building diversified between foxes and hedgehogs? Your success depends upon it.

Chapter 7
Problem Solving

The main reason that decision making is so important is that it is preceded by a problem. Think about it: as a manager, what are you most engaged in? I would bet that it is in solving problems. And lots of problems at that. So often, I will hear a manager say, "I was so busy putting out fires today that I didn't even get to the things on my list." Let me rephrase: "I was so busy solving unexpected problems today that I didn't even get to the expected problems on my list." What are the top characteristics of a problem solver? They are:

- Relentless
    - They never give up until the problem is solved.
- Confident
    - No matter how tough it gets, they never lose faith in their ability to solve the problem.
- Imaginative
    - They not only think freely and creatively but imagine that they have already solved the problem.
- Adaptable
    - Things change, and sometimes they change very quickly. Being adaptable means being able to think (and react) on your feet.

- Patient
  - All good things come to those who wait, and solving problems is no different.
- Iconoclastic
  - They attack established beliefs or institutions.

I can spend hours and days and sometimes weeks trying to figure out the solution to a math or a programming problem. I can tell you with confidence that it took me over a year to finally solve the problem of risk-adjusting claims data to develop our risk-based auditing application. And I mean working at it almost every day. I know many people do not tend to put sustained effort toward solving problems, much less a year to solve one problem. Once the problem-solving muscle starts to get a workout, it becomes enjoyable to be able to exercise it for more sustained periods on bigger and bigger problems.

Maybe the impediment is that we harken back to the day of story problems in middle school, and we start to feel nauseous. Remember those? "Adrianna has 10 pieces of gum to share with her friends. There wasn't enough gum for all her friends, so she went to the store to get 3 more pieces of gum. How many pieces of gum does Adrianna have now?" The answer? Who cares? And who has that many friends, anyway? Maybe I'm a freak, but I *loved* these types of story problems. I have several books on my shelf, that I look at regularly, filled with these types of problems. Let's agree on this: if you do something regularly, eventually you will become good at it, so if you practice formal problem solving on a regular basis, you will become a good problem solver. The prior chapter on "Predicting Like a Pro" involved lots of great problem-solving techniques, and we can apply those to other problems that we may face.

Maybe the best way to start is to just jump right to solving some problems and see how more complex problems are solved.

The Monty Hall Problem

The following narrative is widely available on the internet, although I have never been able to find any specific attribution, so let's proceed on the assumption that it is fair use.

There is a classic mathematical nuisance known as the Monty Hall problem, which can be hard to wrap the mind around. It references the classic game show *Let's Make a Deal*, where a contestant chose one of three doors, knowing that a valuable prize waited behind one, and worthless prizes behind the others.

On the show, once the contestant made their choice, Monty Hall (the host) opened one of the *other* doors, revealing one of the worthless prizes. He would then open the contestant's chosen door to reveal whether they picked correctly. The *Monty Hall problem* asks, "What if the contestant could change her door choice after she saw the worthless prize? Would it be to her advantage to switch doors?" In other words, if the contestant guesses that the new car lay behind door number one, and Monty opened door number two to reveal a goat, is the new car more likely to be behind door number one or door number three?

At this point, the confusion begins to settle in. The most basic understanding is that revealing the contents of one of the other doors simply changed the contestant's odds from 1:3 to 1:2. But that isn't the case. It has been mathematically proven that if the contestant could switch her door to number three after seeing the goat behind number two, she'd be *twice as likely* to win. How can this be? It isn't intuitive, but it's true. Great mathematicians have puzzled over this, as well as great scientists at Los Alamos and professors at MIT.

The best way to look at it is to imagine that, when the contestant selects a door, she divides the doors into two sets: (A) The doors she *did* select, and (B) the doors she did *not* select. At this point, each individual door has a 1:3 chance of being the winning door, but the two *sets* have differing odds. Set A has a 1:3 chance of containing the new car, but Set B, having twice as many doors in it, is twice as likely to contain the winner.

When Monty opens one of the doors in Set B to show it isn't the winner, Set B *still* has a two-in-three chance of holding the winner. The only difference is that there is only one door with unknown contents, so the 2/3 odds go to the unopened door in Set B, while Set A still has it's 1/3 odds. So, revealing the contents of door number two didn't make the contestant's odds any worse, but it did make the odds for door number three improve. Remember, nothing has changed except for our knowledge of what is behind one of the doors. If the game started with only two doors, then the odds would be 1:2, but that was not the case. We started with three doors, and we still have three doors, no matter how much information we have. The other thing to remember is this: Monty does not open the door at random. He knows where the goat is and where the car is. Imagine how anticlimactic it would be if you picked door number one and Monty opened door number two (at random) and there sat the car. Game over!

In explaining the effect, it helps to increase the scale of the question. Imagine that there are 100 doors to choose from instead of three. The contestant chooses a door, and then the host opens 98 other doors to show that they don't contain prizes. Which is more likely to hold the prize…the door she selected initially, or the one door left unopened from the 99 she didn't choose? The answer is much more obvious: the door she chose still has a 1/100 chance of being the winning door, where the other closed door has a 99/100 chance.

The problem is that the human brain is hard-wired to seek out patterns, discarding much of the non-patterned data. This system usually works very well in keeping unimportant information from overwhelming the mind, but occasionally too much information ends up on the cutting-room floor.

Problem Solving

For those that doubt the science, here is incontrovertible evidence that the model does, in fact, work. The more you play the game, the more the ratios move to their actual values. This is a *Monte Carlo simulation*. For example, with 150 players, those who stayed with their original decision won between 25% and 41% of the time. For those that switched, they won between 59% and 74% of the time. When you get to 6,000 players, those who stayed won between 32% and 35% of the time while those that switched won between 65% and 68% of the time.

# of Players	If All Players Switched		If No Player Switched	
	95% Confidence Interval	Expected Value	95% Confidence Interval	Expected Value
9	3-9	6	0-5	3
51	27-40	34	10-23	17
99	57-75	66	24-42	33
150	88-111	100	38-61	50
201	120-146	134	54-80	67
249	151-180	166	68-97	83
300	183-215	200	83-115	100
399	246-283	266	115-152	133
501	313-354	334	146-187	167
999	636-694	666	304-362	333
2001	1293-1375	1334	626-708	667
3000	1949-2051	2000	949-1051	1000
3999	2608-2724	2666	1275-1391	1333
5001	3269-3399	3334	1602-1732	1667
6000	3928-4072	4000	1928-2072	2000

TABLE 7.1   Monte Carlo simulation

I will point out that this is why I don't trust intuition for solving problems or making decisions. Again, it is good for pointing us in the right direction but if you asked 6,000 players whether they would like to stay or switch, the vast majority of them would elect to stay, thereby halving the likelihood of winning the car.

115

The Birthday Paradox

If I asked how many people would it take for the chance that at least 2 people had the same birthday (month and year) to be even, or 50%, most would say 183 people, since this is half of the number of days in a given year, which makes logical sense. The fact is, it only takes 23 people in the same room to have a probability of 50% that at least 2 share the same birthday. At 70 people, the probability it 99.9%. Let's look at how this works, and, to do so, we should start at the beginning. Because we are attempting to pair off people in the room, we need at least 2 people for the calculations. With 1 person, the chances of being born on any day of the year is 365/365, or 1. The chances that the second person is born on the same day is only 1/365, and since we want both of these to happen at the same time, we multiply them together, like this:

$$\frac{365}{365} \cdot \frac{1}{365} = 0.0027$$

FIGURE 7.1   One birthday calculation

Therefore, you have about a 1/400 chance that, if you randomly walked up to a stranger, the 2 of you would share the same birthday. Not great odds, for sure. But what about 4 people? There would be 11 different ways that 2 of these 4 could share the same birthday, and we would have to calculate the probability for each pair, which is a bit of a task. Imagine what it would be like with 25 people!

An easier way is to calculate the *complement*, or the opposite of the question. In other words, we want to ask the likelihood that 2 out of the 4 people in the room *do not* share a birthday. Because this is a probability problem, we know that the total of all the possible results will always be equal to 1, or a 100% chance of occurrence. Rather than calculating how *likely* it is that 2 people would share the same birthday, we calculate how *unlikely* it is, then subtract that from 1 or the 100% chance of occurrence. Looking at the example above with 2 people, the

Problem Solving

complement would be (365/365 * 364/365), or 0.9973, meaning that there is a 99.73% chance that there is *not* a match. If we ran this out for four people, it would look like this:

$$\frac{365}{365} \times \frac{364}{365} \times \frac{363}{365} \times \frac{362}{365} \times = 98.36\%$$

FIGURE 7.2 Four birthdays calculation

Remember, to calculate the chances that they *do* share a birthday, we subtract the results from 1, so, in a room of 4, the chances of sharing a birthday is (1 - 0.9836), or 1.64%. But because we are dealing in exponents, the chances grow quite quickly. By the time we get to 10 people in the same place, the probability that none of them share a birthday is just over 88%, which means the chances that they *do* share a birthday is around 22%. If we were to continue in this way, it would start to get a bit messy, so we resort to the use of factorials, which is a lesson for another day. The good news is that, if you learn how to do that, you could easily get the results for any number of people using a scientific calculator. This graph shows how the exponential growth of both matching and non-matching occurs:

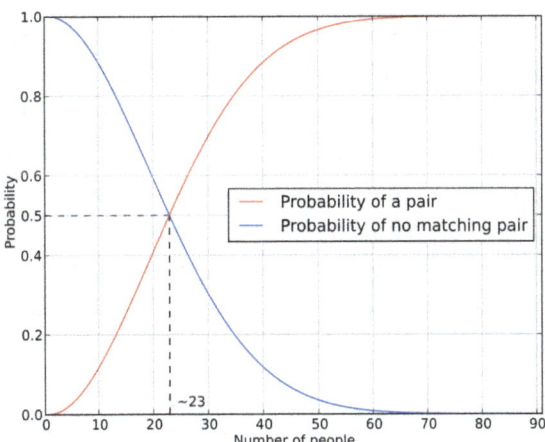

FIGURE 7.2 Matching and non-matching birthdays probability graph

Let's look at a real application for this problem. So far, there have been 44 different presidents of the United States. Donald Trump is the 45th U.S. President, but Grover Cleveland is counted twice because he was elected for two non-consecutive terms. This gives us 946 pairs of birthdays [(44*43)/2], which means that the likelihood of at least two of these presidents having the same birthday is 92.54%. When you check this out, you find that the 11th President of the United States, James K. Polk, was born on November 2, 1795, and that the 29th President, Warren G. Harding, was born on November 2, 1865.

I think the most relevant point here is that these types of solutions are counterintuitive. It doesn't make sense that it only takes 23 people to have a 50% chance of a repeated birthday. And I think that the closer we come to understanding the role that evidence plays in problem solving, as well as in decision making, the closer we come to significantly improving our skills at both.

The Census Problem

One of my favorite problems to teach is the Census problem. That's because the math is not overly difficult but requires a bit of logical thinking to get through. It goes like this:

> A census taker approach is a house and asks the woman who answers the door, "How many children do you have and what are their ages?" The woman responds, "I have 3 children, and the product of their ages is 36." The census taker says, "I need more information than that." The woman replies, "Okay, I would tell you the sum of their ages, but that would confuse you even more." In one last attempt, the census taker asks for any other hint and the woman replies, "My oldest daughter likes cats."

The question is, what are the ages of each of these 3 children? Let's begin by just applying a bit of logic. First, what is it mean "that the product of their ages is 36?" It means that if you multiply the three ages together, they would equal 36. So, from a practical standpoint, how

Problem Solving

many different ways can you multiply three sets of numbers together to get 36? The answer is 8. For example, 1×1×36 = 36. Or 1×3×12 = 36. Or 2×3×6 = 36. So, the way to begin would be to put together a table that shows all the products of three numbers that would equal 36. If we did that, it would look something like this:

Daughter 1	Daughter 2	Daughter 3
1	1	36
1	2	18
1	3	12
1	4	9
1	6	6
2	2	9
2	3	6
3	3	4

TABLE 7.2   Three daughters' ages table

Now that we have all the components, let's go to the next clue. The woman says, "I would tell you the sum of their ages, but that would confuse you even more." We'll add a column to the table where we calculate that and see what we get.

Look closely at this table in the last column. Are there any values that are confusing? Look closely at the 5th and the 6th set of three: 1 + 6 + 6 = 13 and 2 + 2 + 9 = 13. If the woman had told the census taker that the sum of their ages was 13, he would've still faced a dilemma because there are two sums equal to 13. Therefore, the answer must be one of those two sets of three ages. Now let's look at the last clue. The woman says, "My oldest daughter likes cats." Therefore, of the three numbers, one of them—and only one of them—must be larger than the other two. That only occurs in the set of 2, 2, and 9, because, in the other set, there is a match for the two larger numbers (both have a value of 6) and therefore would not fulfill the third clue. So, in this case, as a

Daughter 1	Daughter 2	Daughter 3	Sum
1	1	36	38
1	2	18	21
1	3	12	16
1	4	9	14
1	6	6	13
2	2	9	13
2	3	6	11
3	3	4	10

TABLE 7.3 Three daughters' ages with sum table

solution to the problem, the daughters' ages are two years old, two years old and nine years old.

Strategies for Problem Solving

In a blog entry called "Using Psychology" on October 15, 2019, Professor John Malouff of the University of New England, Armidale, Australia, contributed a great post with over fifty problem-solving strategies explained in detail. Some of these we have already discussed, but I found all of them to be very applicable and helpful. For purposes of brevity, I did not include them all, so I recommend you go to the following link noted in the endnotes to review all the strategies, along with a more detailed description of each.

Strategies to Help You Understand the Problem:

- Clarify the problem.
- Identify key elements of the problem.
- Visualize the problem or a relevant process or situation.
- Draw a picture or diagram of the problem or relevant process or situation.
- Create a model of the problem or a relevant process.
- Imagine being the problem, a key process, or the solution.

- Simulate or act out a key element of the problem.
- Consider a specific example.
- Consider extreme cases.
- Acquire knowledge of relevant domains.
- Change perspective.
- Consider levels and systems.

Strategies to Help You Simplify the Task:

- Solve one part at a time.
- Redefine the problem.

Strategies to Help You Determine the Cause of a Problem:

- Collect information about what happens before, during, and after the problem.
- Organize information into a table, chart, or list and look for a pattern.
- Try to make the problem worse.
- Compare situations with and without the problem.
- Consider multiple causes and interactions.
- Consider nonlinear effects.

Strategies Involving the Use of External Aids to Help You Identify Possible Solutions:

- Ask someone, especially an expert.
- Seek the answer and written material.
- Use a tool or technology.
- Apply a theory.
- Apply the scientific method.
- Use mathematics.
- Use a formula.

And Finally, Strategies to Help You Function Optimally while Problem-Solving:

- Think of options without immediately evaluating them.
- Set a goal with a purpose you value.
- Avoid distraction.
- Work in a new setting.
- Adjust time limit to optimum.
- Work with someone else.
- Create a positive mood with an optimum arousal level.
- Think of the problem is a challenge or opportunity.
- Think confidently.
- Take a break.
- Persist.

Dr. Malouff includes a few references:

- D'Zurilla, T.J., & Goldfried, M.R. (1971). Problem solving and behaviour modification. Journal of Abnormal Psychology, 78, 104–126.
- Fabian, J. (1990). Creative thinking & problem solving. Chelsea, MI:Lewis.
- Harris, R. (2002). *Problem solving techniques.*
- McNamara, C. (1999). *Basic guidelines to problem solving and decision making.*

CHAPTER 8

Process Improvement as a Composite Model

So far, what we have three critical concepts for the evidence-based model:

- Evidence
  - in the form of data and other information
- Decision making
  - using that evidence
- Problem solving
  - as an application of evidence-based decision making.

Intuitively, it feels like we have all the pieces to our puzzle. But then, you know how I feel about intuition. What we are missing is a platform that we can use to implement all these tools that we've learned and, in my opinion, the best platforms are found within the process improvement arena. In particular, Lean Six Sigma. There are many books written on this topic, and, in fact, I have written and published one. The purpose here is not to teach you how to become a subject matter expert in Lean Six Sigma, but rather introduce the idea of using it as a platform to bring these three critical concepts together and apply them to solve practical problems within our organizations.

In its holistic approach, Lean Six Sigma is all about efficiency. But before it gets to that point, it's really about evidence-based management. The first step in the process is *classification*. This is really about discovery; learning about what's going on around us to help us define the problem. The first step in making a decision (or solving a problem or managing a situation) is to identify what it is that we're looking at. In classification, we want to ask ourselves three basic questions:

- What do we see?
- What did we find or discover?
- How does it work?

At its core, we are trying to identify the issue and get a better idea of its inner workings and what surrounds it by using the classification technique. In fact, this helps us to identify what kind of a problem it might be. Maybe it involves an issue with physical space, determining whether some capital improvement project is needed. Or maybe it has to do with reducing costs or improving efficiencies in some process within the organization. Or even converting some manual processes to automated processes using technology. This might include an e-prescribing system or an EHR component or dealing with impediments within our revenue cycle process.

The second technique has to do with *correlation* or creating a better understanding of the relationships between issues. Again, we want to ask ourselves three questions:

- Are the events related?
- How are they related?
- How strong is that relationship

From a technical perspective, correlation is a mathematical conclusion and is often confused with concepts of simple association. If we measure or quantify those relationships, we are using correlation. But in some cases, we might infer the strength of an association to get an idea of whether the issues are even related to each other. In correlation, we calculate the relationship on a scale that ranges between -1 and 1.

At either end of the scale, the relationship is equally strong, but a negative correlation indicates an inverse relationship, while a positive correlation indicates a reciprocal relationship. For example, as the cost of doing business increases, profitability decreases. This is an example of a negative correlation. An example of a positive correlation would be that the more office visits a provider encounters produces, the more work RVUs reported. Let's say we have a dramatic shift in our payer mix and at the same time experience a change in our revenue. We could easily measure that to determine both the magnitude and the direction of that relationship. Perhaps the most important thing to remember about this is that even though two or more events may be correlated, one may not cause the other. Which brings me to our third technique: *causation*.

It's been my experience that when organizations have struggled with solving problems that they know our problems, it's because they didn't get to this step of cause and effect. Think how difficult it is to fix something if you don't know what broke it. This is true for every industry, not just healthcare. And it applies to our personal as well as our professional lives. All we are trying to do here is link together different events. And to do this, we must ask ourselves some basic questions, such as:

- Does an event in one area cause a change in another area?
- Is there a threshold of that causation?
- Why did it happen?

Establishing causation is a lot more difficult than correlation and often requires that we use quantitative tools. I read once that about half of all accidents occur within five miles of a person's home. So, a potential solution to this problem would be to move. I guess that might be true if you could show a causative relationship between home and the accidents, but the fact is that approximately 82% of all driving occurs within 5 miles of home and, therefore, while it is highly correlated, it is not causal. Or how about this one: of all automobile crashes, the driver of at least one of the vehicles ate within 6 hours of the crash. That's an extremely high correlation. Does that mean that eating causes car accidents? Of course not. In fact, about 90% of people eat within every 6-hour period when they are awake. So, coincidence, but not causation.

If we have a change in our payer mix and a subsequent change in our revenue, we want to know whether one causes the other. Did an increase in our Medicare payer mix cause a decrease in our revenue? Or were there other confounding variables? Maybe loss of a provider or two. Maybe a change in payment policies on some other payer. Maybe it occurred because we changed our billing system. How about lead time to appointment and no-shows? I see this a lot where it may take several weeks for a patient to see a provider within the organization and, the longer it takes, the greater the rate of no-shows. Does one cause the other? I can tell you that in the cases I've studied, it does. There is a definite causal relationship between the time it takes for a patient to see the doctor and the number or rate of no-shows in the office. So, if you want to reduce your no-shows, you reduce the lead time to appointment.

And there's another question we must ask ourselves here: if I fix one problem, does it create another problem in another area? These are *unseen* or *unexpected consequences* and can be devastating to an organization. I will give you an example from my personal archives. My in-laws live in a small town up in the Catskill Mountains of New York. Behind their property is a significant hill, which slopes down through their property, down the road, and then into the Catskill Creek. To control the drainage, my father-in-law had put a small culvert under the driveway to allow the water to pass through into a little creek that ran to the front yard, under a little bridge, and then down to the creek.

One year, many years ago, we had so much rain that the culvert couldn't handle it and it washed away the driveway. So, when we went to repair it, we put in a larger pipe. I calculated the estimated size of that pipe based on our best guess of the volume of water that would pass through it. Several months later, they had a massive rainstorm. And I'm happy to say that it worked; the water got within a couple inches of the top of the culvert, but it did not wash over the driveway. If that was the end of the story, it would've been great news, but it's not. Rather, this larger pipe allowed so much water to flow through that it ended up washing out the front yard and taking out the bridge.

Sometimes the unexpected consequences can be positive. A few years ago, I was working with a practice on a basic process improvement project. The goal was to decrease patient throughput time to allow the practice to see more patients in a given day. This is a classic problem that goes to the importance of efficiency. Doing more with the same results in more profitability. The second point of contact with the patient, after the scheduling process, is the waiting room, a regular point of frustration for patients and medical staff. As is my custom, I sat in the waiting room for several hours just observing the patients and their interactions with the front desk staff during the check-in procedure. I noticed that many of the older new patients would make several trips back up to the front desk to ask questions of the staff. At the end of the first day, I met with the front desk staff and asked them about these additional patient questions. They said there were two primary issues: (1) patients did not understand the financial obligations page, and (2) they couldn't read the print because they had forgotten their reading glasses.

That evening, I went out to a Sam's Club and I purchased twenty reading glasses in different strengths. That next morning, we put those reading glasses into a basket with a sign that said, "If you forgot your reading glasses, feel free to borrow a pair of ours." That step alone reduced the average time it took a new patient to complete the intake form by 7 minutes, which was a nearly 30% reduction in the total time. Resolving that issue helped to reduce overall waiting time enough to allow the practice to see three additional patients a day. At $110 in revenue per patient, this brought an increase in revenues of almost $30,000. Not all consequences are bad.

Here's a common example that I run into all the time. Organizations spend a great deal of time, resources, and money in coding education and training for their providers. What we might want to know is whether that training decreases the risk of noncompliance. Or is it due to some change in policies or guidelines? The answer helps us develop an ROI for that process.

Adopting these principles and techniques won't guarantee that we will always be successful but will guarantee that we will be *more* successful than if we rely on anecdote or brute force alone. I remember, years ago, working with several practices that were looking to get out from under the burden of working with third-party payers. No matter how you look at it, the relationship between providers and payers is adversarial, the degree to which varies depending upon the payers in the market. An obvious solution was for the provider to divorce themselves from all third-party payers and deal directly with the patient. The challenge facing practice administrators is trying to anticipate what the financial repercussions might be from such a move. A third-party payer system had been in place for many decades and most healthcare providers have never had to deal directly with their patients, apart from collecting co-pays and deductibles.

The solution? Let's look at the evidence. In October of 2007, there was an article published in the Journal of Health Economics written by Jonathan Gruber and David Rodriguez, both with the Department of Economics at the Massachusetts Institute of Technology. Some will remember Jonathan Gruber as one of the principle architects of the Affordable Care Act. The title of the article was "How Much Uncompensated Care Do Doctors Provide?" There have been other attempts at this type of analysis prior, but they relied upon list prices for their calculations. The problem is that these list prices would overestimate the true amount of uncompensated care, since in many cases they were inflated to account for the deeply discounted rates being paid by insurance companies at the time.

For example, if an uninsured patient receives a procedure with a list price of $200, but insurance companies only pay $90 on average, we might conclude that the patient received $90 worth of care. If the patient paid nothing, then we call that $90 of uncompensated care. If an uninsured patient pays $200 for a procedure for which an insurance company would've paid $90, then we say that the patient received a $-110 of uncompensated care.

To conduct this study, the authors obtained data from detailed financial records for 3,860 physicians from 317 practices and 60 specialties. This included 4.4 million visits from 1.8 million patients and, of those, 3.9% (162,000) were from uninsured patients. The insurance status was determined by looking at the insurance information that was associated to each claim. Significantly, the sample was not random. It did, however, generate a considerable interest and provided a platform for others to replicate their own studies. I did this on several occasions with providers that were considering abandoning the third-party payer system.

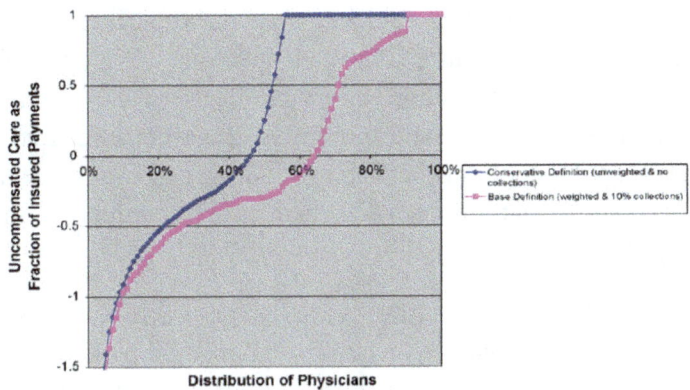

FIGURE 8.1   How much uncompensated care do physicians provide?

In the above graph, a value of 1 means that a doctor received no payments from the uninsured patient. A value of 60 means the uninsured patients paid the same as what insured patients would've paid, and a negative value means the doctor found the uninsured patients more profitable. Between 45% and 59% of physicians provide negative uncompensated care; that is, they collect more, on average, from their uninsured patients than from their insured patients. Between 12% and 14% of physicians found their uninsured patients were more than twice as profitable as their insured patients. How could that be? One reason was because the provider had a reasonable fee schedule, which made a significant impact on the provider success under this model. If you look at how the typical provider creates a fee schedule, it is disproportionately high to accommodate the significant reductions tendered by private payers. Want to get paid $100 for that procedure that costs you $60 to deliver? Charge $200 and hope for the best. In concierge medicine and amongst those providers that have simply dropped commercial insurance, charging a reasonable amount (say, $100 in this case) brings with it a greater likelihood of payment (partially or fully) for the same amount of effort.

If we look at this from the patient perspective, we see that between 35% and 53% of patients receive some uncompensated care. In this study, 26% of patients paid nothing for the care that they received, and the minority of patients paid less than the typical insured patient receiving the same procedure. Between 38% and 52% paid 100% of the list price for the procedure or service. Between 47% and 65% of uninsured patients actually paid more than the average insured patient. And, surprisingly enough, between 8.5% and 9.6% of uninsured patients paid more than double what their insured counterparts paid for the same procedure.

Let's look at this from the physician perspective. For providers, uncompensated care, measured relative to all insured patients, is -0.07% of patient care revenues and 0.59% of patient care revenues using the upper bound estimate. Relative to the privately insured, uncompensated care ranges from 0.24% of revenues to 0.8% of revenues. Relative to Medicaid, uncompensated care ranged from -0.75% of revenues to 0.16% of revenues. Now factor in the cost of doing business with third-party payers, which can include spending up to 14% just to collect what is owed, plus a reduction in compliance risk, and the potential for profitability soars.

Granted, the study was completed in 2007 and much has changed in the last 12 years. But only regarding the numbers, not the challenges. This study used estimated discounting factors of 55% from 2005. Is it a deeper discount now? The study also did not consider the cost to the practice of claims processing. According to a study published in the online *Journal of the American Medical Association* on February 20, 2018, the estimated cost to process a claim for a single patient encounter or event ranged from $20 for primary care visit to $215 for an inpatient surgical procedure. It also found that estimated administrative costs represent 25% to 31% of total health care expenditures in the United States. And of *that*, at least 62%, based on prior studies, is attributed to billing and insurance related activities.

We also have the problem with denials. According to an article published in *Becker's Hospital CFO report* written by Kelly Gooch, an estimated $262 billion of the $3 trillion in claims submitted by hospitals in 2016 were initially denied. This was based on a study reported by Change Healthcare. The study also found that 63% of these denied claims are recoverable on average, but providers have to spend roughly $118 per claim and appeals. If you take all these costs together, which are almost exclusively driven based on relationships with third-party payers, and you were to eliminate these, imagine the increase in profitability and the reduction in the hassle factor associated with being a healthcare provider.

So, do I recommend that every practice should dump their payers and work straight with the patient on financial matters? No. Because it won't work for everyone. Practices that have a lower average rate per service unit would be more successful, since the fee schedules are more easily absorbed by patients who do not have insurance. What I *am* recommending, however, is that each practice conduct payer profitability analyses and make the decision based on their own results, rather than those of someone else.

One of the unexpected consequences of this issue of third-party payer relationships has resulted in a significant increase in concierge medicine in the United States. While we experienced the beginning of this movement in the late 1990s, by 2004, the Government Accountability Office reported that there were 146 such practices in the United States, mostly concentrated on the East and West Coasts. In concierge medicine, sometimes called retainer medicine, patients will pay an annual fee to the physician for a more exclusive access and short notice appointments and phone consultations. In some cases, the retainer fee will cover all such services while in others, the physician will still bill a reasonable amount for individual consultations. The retainer portion is what separates concierge medicine from practices that deal directly with the patient financially, but do not charge a retainer. How is it working? Well, in 2012, the Physician's Foundation reported that there were 4,400 private physicians participating in concierge-based medicine.

This issue is the poster child for critical thinking and evidence-based management in healthcare. In the end, for the typical healthcare manager and administrator, there is a lot to figure out. From a collaboration perspective, we must look at developing products and services with physicians, which often means developing successful and workable joint ventures. To do this, we must pursue joint contracting arrangements and share development of strategic plans and budgets. We must be able to coexist with all our providers by investing and supporting selected initiatives. A terrific way to do this is to expand provider participation in management and governmental affairs. I know there are a lot of people who tell me that there is no way that they want physicians involved in management or administration, and I will tell you that I believe they are dead wrong. Physicians are not only smart, but they are passionate about what they do. And smart and passionate are two key characteristics to successful leaders.

With the changing healthcare reimbursement system, we must be able to make sure that we can develop favorable physician reimbursement models with system-owned health plans and resist initiatives perceived as threatening to the providers' interests. From a standpoint of competition, particularly if you're working in an integrated delivery system or a larger health system, acquiring specialty and primary care practices is a huge objective. With turnover, we must regularly recruit and employ replacement physicians, and with that, leverage payer relationships to maximize provider and hospital payments. And finally, include our providers and hospital-owned and freestanding ancillary ambulatory services.

In Closing

Set theory can be defined as the branch of mathematics that deals with the formal properties of sets as units (without regard to the nature of their individual constituents) and the expression of other branches of mathematics in terms of sets. A theory formally introduced by Georg Cantor, a German mathematician (1845-1918), it is broadly about treating infinite sets as mathematical objects that could be considered in the same way that we consider (or construct) finite sets. Set theory helped to revolutionize mathematics in general, while also specifically impacting the design of digital electronic circuitry and hence, the development and improvement of personal computers.

But for every one of these theories, there is a paradox. For set theory, that paradox is the Barber's Paradox, which goes like this: "The barber is the one who shaves all those, and only those, who do not shave themselves." The question is, does the barber shave himself? The paradox is, if the barber does shave himself then he can't shave himself, because he only shaves those who do not shave themselves, so if he does, then he can't. The question is whether the barber can be in the set of those who don't shave themselves if he does, in fact, shave himself. I know it sounds silly, and seems like just semantics, but by probing the nature of the definitions of the data, the barber paradox forces us to question the application of every theory—in every situation.

Remember, our lives are steeped in uncertainty. The evidence around us is no difference. We are faced with uncertainties, paradoxes and incomplete facts. In colloquial terms, Godel's Second Incompleteness Theorem states that any formal system that is interesting enough to formulate its own consistency can prove its own consistency if it is inconsistent. What? Basically, Godel proved that with any given mathematical system, there will always be certain statements that cannot be proven within the system. In essence, he posits that there will always be some things that are improvable and incomplete, even in the field of mathematics. As it applies to us and this book, we need to accept the fact that, no matter how hard we try and no matter how much evidence we have, there will be decisions we have to make that will be based as much on our critical thinking and judgment as they will on the evidence and the data. Morris Kline, a 20th century mathematician and philosopher, wrote the following on the work of Kurt Godel: "The one distinguishing feature of mathematics that it might have claimed in this century, is that the absolute certainty of its results could no longer be claimed."

I believe that this idea of uncertainty is best illustrated by Bertrand Russell in this famous quote:

> I wanted certainty in the kind of way that people want religious faith. I thought that certainty is most likely to be found in mathematics than elsewhere. But I discovered that many mathematical demonstrations that my teachers expected me to accept were full of fallacies and that, if certainty were indeed discoverable in mathematics, it would be in a new field of mathematics with more solid foundations than those that had hitherto thought secure. But as the work proceeded, I was continually reminded of the fable of the elephant and the tortoise. Having constructed an elephant upon which the mathematical world could rest, I found the elephant tottering and proceeded to construct a tortoise to keep the elephant from falling. But the tortoise was not more secure than the elephant. And after some 20 years of arduous toil, I came to the conclusion that there was nothing more that I could do in the way of making mathematical knowledge indubitable.[49]

When I read this for the first time, it broke my heart. Being a lifelong mathematician, an obsessive-compulsive mathematician, I had always believed that mathematics paved the way for absolute truth and

In Closing

brought truth to power through that absoluteness. But now, I know that is not the case. There is an absolute truth, but that is for another day. It just means that we do the best we can with what we have, and I can accept that. "Work the problem," is what I was taught as a corpsman in the Navy. That simply meant that to stop, take a breath, look around, identify the available tools, then do the next right thing. Life is all about solving problems—every day, in oftentimes new, exciting, and even scary ways. Evidence-based practice is all about making decisions, which is all about solving those problems. If we can do nothing more than minimize the uncertainty around those decisions, we have, in fact, worked the problem.

I hope that this book has provided you with the tools necessary to improve the outcomes of your management decisions and to help increase the success of your projects. It is my hope that, if nothing else, you adopted the mantra, "We will no longer make decisions without data." I believe that I can sum up my thoughts best with the quote from Jeffrey Pfeffer and Robert Sutton based on an article they wrote on evidence-based management in the *Harvard Business Review*. It goes like this:

> Facts and evidence are great levelers of hierarchy. Evidence-based practice changes power dynamics, replacing formal authority, reputation, and intuition with data. This means that senior leaders—often venerated for their wisdom and decisiveness—may lose some stature as their intuitions are replaced, at least at times, by judgments based on data available to virtually any educated person. The implication is that leaders need to make a fundamental decision: Do they want to be told they are always right, or do they want to lead organizations that actually perform well?[50]

So, don't just do something, stand there!

Reference Notes and Resources

1 Tom Feilden, "Most of Scientists 'Can't Replicate Studies by Their Peers,'" BBC News, February 22, 2017, https://www.bbc.com/news/science-environment-39054778.

2 Monya Baker, "1,500 Scientists Lift the Lid on Reproducibility," *Nature*, May 25, 2016, corrected July 28, 2016, https://www.nature.com/news/1-500-scientists-lift-the-lid-on-reproducibility-1.19970.

3 Joint Statistical Meetings 2017, Baltimore, MD.

4 Isaiah Berlin, *The Hedgehog and the Fox: An Essay on Tolstoy's View of History*. Princeton University Press.

5 Ibid.

6 Jim Collins, *Good to Great: Why Some Companies Make the Leap and Others Don't*. HarperBusiness.

7 Isaiah Berlin.

8 Jim Collins.

9 Kristof, Nicholas, "Learning How to Think," *The New York Times*, March 26, 2009, https://www.nytimes.com/2009/03/26/opinion/26Kristof.html.

10 Malcolm Gladwell, *Blink: The Power of Thinking Without Thinking*, Little, Brown and Company; 1st edition. January 11, 2005. 288 pp.

11 Edgar Allan Poe, Edgar Allan, "The System of Dr. Tarr and Professor Fether," (1856), accessed April 13, 2019, https://poestories.com/read/systemoftarr.

12 "National Academy of Sciences Releases Landmark Report on Memory and Eyewitness Identification, Urges Reform of Police Identification Procedures," The Innocence Project, accessed April 24, 2019, https://www.innocenceproject.org/national-academy-of-sciences-releases-landmark-report-on-memory-and-eyewitness-identification-urges-reform-of-police-identification-procedures/.

13 Grissinger, Matthew, "Rapid Response Teams in Hospitals Increase Patient Safety." *Pharmacy and Therapeutics,* April 2010, https://www.ncbi.nlm.nih.gov/pmc/articles/PMC2873718/.

14 Ibid.

15 "Rapid Response Teams: The Case for Early Intervention," *Improvement Stories,* Institute for Healthcare Improvement, accessed June 11, 2019, http://www.ihi.org/resources/Pages/ImprovementStories/RapidResponseTeamsTheCaseforEarlyIntervention.aspx.

16 Frédéric Brochet & Gil Morrot, "Influence of the Context on the Perception of Wine Cognitive and Methodological Implications," *Journal International des Sciences de la Vigne et du Vin,* 1999, http://oeno-one.eu/article/view/1017.

17 William Ely Hill, "My Wife and My Mother-in-Law," *Puck Magazine,* November 6, 1915, http://www.loc.gov/pictures/item/2010652001/.

18 Source: https://dumielauxepices.net/sites/default/files/optical-illusion-clipart-duck-rabbit-702181-1862513.png

19 Jeffrey Pfeffer and Robert I. Sutton, "Evidence-Based Management," *Harvard Business Review,* January 2006, https://hbr.org/2006/01/evidence-based-management.

20 Source: http://www.businessdictionary.com/definition/law-of-diminishing-returns.html, accessed April 14, 2019.

21 Barbara J. Sahakian and Jamie Nicole LaBuzetta, *Bad Moves: How Decision Making Goes Wrong, and the Ethics of Smart Drugs*, Oxford University Press, May 8, 2013.

22 Brian Wansink and Jeffery Sobal, "Mindless Eating: The 200 Daily Food Decisions We Overlook," *Environment and Behavior,* January 2007, available at SSRN: https://ssrn.com/abstract=2710887.

23 Joel Hoomans, "35,000 Decisions: The Great Choices of Strategic Leaders," *Leading Edge Journal,* Mar 20, 2015, https://go.roberts.edu/leadingedge/the-great-choices-of-strategic-leaders.

24 "7 Steps to Effective Decision Making," University of Massachusetts Dartmouth, accessed June 11, 2019, https://www.umassd.edu/media/umassdartmouth/fycm/decision_making_process.pdf.

25 Herbert Simon, *Administrative Behavior: A Study of Decision-Making Processes in Administrative Organizations,* (1947) MacMillan, New York.

26 Ibid.

27 Randall Bartlett, *Economic Foundations of Political Power* (1973) Free Press, New York, 1973, from Chapter 2.

28 "List of Cognitive Biases: Decision-Making, Belief, and Behavioral Biases," *Wikipedia.org,* accessed June 11, 2019, https://en.wikipedia.org/wiki/List_of_cognitive_biases#Decision-making,_belief,_and_behavioral_biases.

29 William Shakespeare, *As You Like It,* Act 5, Scene 1.

30 Bertrand Russell, *New Hopes for a Changing World,* (1951).

31 James Chen, reviewer, "Sunk Cost Trap," *Investopedia.com,* April 18, 2018. https://www.investopedia.com/terms/s/sunk-cost-trap.asp.

32 "Quick Safety 28: Cognitive Biases in Health Care," The Joint Commission, Division of Health Care Improvement, October 25, 2016, https://www.jointcommission.org/issues/article.aspx?Article=cqF0HgDFcsy4VsiyOztvk7%2bOSJL0abm67PQ7hjWn4PI%3d.

33 Michael Shermer, "Wrong Again: Why Experts' Predictions Fail, Especially About the Future," *Huffington Post,* January 5, 2012, https://www.huffpost.com/entry/wrong-again-why-experts-p_b_1181657.

34 Hugh Courtney, et al., "Strategy under uncertainty," *Harvard Business Review,* November-December 1997, pp. 66-79, available at https://hbr.org/1997/11/strategy-under-uncertainty.

35 Clifford Chi, "Rational Decision Making: The 7-Step Process for Making Logical Decisions," *Hubspot Blog,* updated April 17 2019 https://blog.hubspot.com/marketing/rational-decision-making

36 Pascal's wager: "And so our proposition is of infinite force, when there is the finite to stake in a game where there are equal risks of gain and of loss, and the infinite to gain. This is demonstrable; and if men are capable of any truths, this is one."

37 Heidi D. Nelson, "Screening for Breast Cancer: An Update for the U.S. Preventive Services Task Force," *Annals of Internal Medicine,* November 17,

2009, accessed June 11, 2019, https://annals.org/aim/fullarticle/745247/screening-breast-cancer-update-u-s-preventive-services-task-force.

38 Mei-Sing Ong and Kenneth D. Mandl, "National Expenditure for False-Positive Mammograms and Breast Cancer Overdiagnoses Estimated at $4 Billion a Year" *Health Affairs*, April 2015, https://www.researchgate.net/publication/274644646_National_Expenditure_For_False-Positive_Mammograms_And_Breast_Cancer_Overdiagnoses_Estimated_At_4_Billion_A_Year.

39 Harold C. Sox, et al. *Medical Decision Making*, Boston: Butterworth (1988) available at https://www.academia.edu/7080354/Medical_Decision_Making_2nd_ed.

40 Jeremiah A. Barondess, Harvey A. McGehee, Charles C. J. Carpenter, editors, *Differential Eiagnosis*, Philadelphia: Lea & Febiger (1994).

41 Erin P. Balogh, Bryan T. Miller, and John R. Ball, editors, *Improving Diagnosis in Health Care*, National Academies of Sciences, Engineering, and Medicine; Institute of Medicine; Board on Health Care Services; Committee on Diagnostic Error in Health Care (2015).

42 Jane Weaver, "More People Search for Health Online," *Telemedicine on NBCNews.com*, July 16, 2013, http://www.nbcnews.com/id/3077086/t/more-people-search-health-online/#.XLPqf-hKiUk.

43 John Malouff, "Over Fifty Problem-Solving Strategies Explained," *Using Psychology (blog)*, October 15, 2018, https://blog.une.edu.au/usingpsychology/2018/10/15/over-fifty-problem-solving-strategies-explained/.

44 Thomas J. D'Zurilla and Marvin R. Goldfried, "Problem Solving and Behavior Modification," *Journal of Abnormal Psychology*, August 1971, available at https://psycnet.apa.org/buy/1972-02205-001.

45 John Fabian, *Creative Thinking & Problem Solving*, Chelsea, MI:Lewis (1990).

46 Robert A. Harris, *Creative Problem Solving: A Step-By-Step Approach*, Pyrczak Publishing (2002).

47 Carter McNamara, "Basic Guidelines to Problem Solving and Decision Making," 1999, https://www.uaa.alaska.edu/academics/college-of-health/departments/center-for-human-development/Reducing-Recidivism-Conference/_documents/problem-solving.pdf.

48 Jonathan Gruber and David Rodriguez, "How Much Uncompensated Care Do Doctors Provide?" The National Bureau of Economic Research (NBER), *NBER Working Paper No. 13585*, November 2007, available at https://www.nber.org/papers/w13585.

49 Bertrand Russell, 'Reflections on My Eightieth Birthday, *'Portraits from Memory* (1956), pp 54.

50 Jeffrey Pfeffer and Robert Sutton.

Glossary

Term	Definition
Ambiguous stimuli	Illusions that are open to interpretation.
Ashby's Law of Requisite Variety	"The larger the variety of actions available to a control system, the larger the variety of perturbations it is able to compensate." Ashby 1958, 83ff
Asymmetry of information (see also, rational ignorance)	A situation where one person or party has more or better information that another person or party. The information that we have, whether in the form of data or evidence or other materials, often comes from a source that has an incentive to use the information under their control to try to influence our decisions.
Attribute appraisal (see also, variable appraisal)	In an attribute appraisal, we measure each event as a pass/fail. There is no gray area.
Availability bias	The tendency to make decisions or form opinions based o n the information that is readily available or comes most easily to mind. Also called *availability heuristic*.
Average (see also, mean)	The average is the most common that people tend to use but also the most inappropriate metric in the types of distributions we encounter in healthcare. The mean adds up all of the values in the set of numbers and then divides the sum by the number of data points.
Blivet	An image that diplays two irreconcilable images at once. Impossible trident and five-legged elephant are two examples.
Bounded rationality	Decision-making that favors subjectivity, intuition, and anecdote, because only so much information can be gathered and then brought to bear upon a decision.

Causation [In Lean Six Sigma]	A technique to determine what the real causes of a problem are.
Central tendency	For the purposes of this book, this includes, the mean, the median, and the mode.
Classification [In Lean Six Sigma]	A technique to identify what's going on around us to help properly define the problem.
Cognitive diversity (see also, heuristic diversity)	A measurement of how different the rules that people on a team use to make decisions and solve problems.
Complement	The opposite of the question. For instance, instead of asking how many more of one aspect of a calculation, reverse it and ask how many fewer of the inverse aspect.
Concierge medicine (see also, retainer medicine)	Patients pay an annual fee to the physician for more exclusive access and short-notice appointments and phone consultations. In some cases, the retainer fee will cover all such services, while, in others, the physician will still bill a reasonable amount for individual consultations.
Confirmation bias	The tendency to interpret new evidence (or look for existing evidence and information) that confirms our pre-existing theories, these, or beliefs.
Correlation [In Lean Six Sigma]	A technique to create a better understanding of the relationships between issues.
Distribution	A distribution is a visualization of what the data look like when plotted on a graph.
Diversity Prediction Theorem	A diverse crowd will always be more accurate than a single individual or its average member.

Glossary

Dunning-Kruger effect	A cognitive bias where poor performers imagine their abilities are greater than they are. They are unable to learn from their mistakes because they are unaware they are making them. The same lack of competence that causes them to make poor performance choices also impedes their ability to understand they are performing poorly.
Extrapolation method	An estimation of the value based on extending unknown sequence of values or facts be on the area that is certainly known.
Framing bias	Describes a bias that develops from how information is framed or how it is presented. (Not to be confused with *framing effect*.
Heuristic diversity (see also, cognitive diversity)	A measurement of how different the rules that people on a team use to make decisions and solve problems.
Heuristics	Rules that people use to make decisions and solve problems.
Linear decomposition	Relies upon the ability to deconstruct (or decompose) an aggregate whole into its component parts so that the value of the parts together equal or approximate the value of the whole.
Mean (see also, average)	The mean is the most common measure that people tend to use, but it is also the most inappropriate metric in the types of distributions we encounter in healthcare. The mean adds up all of the values in the set of numbers and then divides the sum by the number of data points.
Measures of error or estimation	For the purposes of this book, this includes the covariance, correlation, and regression

Measures of location (see also, central tendency)	For the purposes of this book, this includes, the mean, the median, and the mode.
Measures of variation or dispersion	For the purposes of this book, this includes, the mean, the median, and the mode.
Median	The median assesses data points by location, rather than value.
Mode	The mode is the value that shows up the most. This is determined by sorting the frequency for the value of interest in either ascending or descending order. The value that has the highest frequency is considered the mode.
Monte Carlo simulation	The more you play the game, the more the ratios move to their actual values.
Nash equilibrium	In game theory, when each player knows what the other player's strategy is and no one play has an incentive to change their strategy for personal gain.
Overconfidence effect	A cognitive bias where we are more confident in our judgments or decisions than objective assessment would support. Sometimes called *overconfidence bias.*
Pascal's Wager	And so our proposition is of infinite force, when there is the finite to stake in a game where there are equal risks of gain and of loss, and the infinite to gain. This is demonstrable; and if men are capable of any truths, this is one.
Percentile	The percentile or percentile ranking represents the location of the data point compared to all other data points. Not to be confused with percentage.
Precision	Refers to how close estimates from different samples are to each other.

Glossary

Prediction by Analogy	Estimating the value of a given entity based on similar values in a different entity.
Prediction horizon	Define how far ahead the model can predict the future.
Probe audits	A strategy that hopes to identify risk by pulling charts at random to audit for compliance. An example of anecdotal management.
Rational ignorance (see also, asymmetry of information)	Asymmetry of information occurs because we have determined that the cost of obtaining the information is greater than the benefit of what we might learn. Therefore, it becomes a irrational to waste time and money and resources to gain that information.
Red panda effect	Seeing what you expect or want to see.
Remotely conscious decisions	Decisions that are almost automatic.
Retainer medicine (see also, concierge medicine)	Patients pay an annual fee to the physician for more exclusive access and short-notice appointments and phone consultations. In some cases, the retainer fee will cover all such services, while, in others, the physician will still bill a reasonable amount for individual consultations.
Risk	Assess the likelihood that an outcome will result in some loss to the system.
Risk-based auditing	Use of data and analytics to generate predictive models that assess the likelihood that a billing/coding audit will occur and which specific providers and/or procedures are the most likely targets.

Sampling error	Because the sample is never identical to the population from which it was drawn, if we use the sample to measure the results of that sample and don't infer it to the population, then we are fine. But if we are going to use the results to try to estimate what the entire population looks like, we must account for that error.
Scalar	Compared to a vector with magnitude and direction (see below), a scalar is described by its magnitude only.
Scenario method	Visualizing what future conditions or events are probable as well as what their consequences or effects would be like and how to respond and/or benefit from them.
Strategies	Long-term objectives or global plans for an organization or individual.
Sunk cost bias	The "tendency for people to irrationally follow through on an activity that is not meeting their expectations because of the time and/or money they have already invested." [Investopedia.com] Sometimes called the *sunk cost fallacy* or the *sunk cost trap*.
Tactics	Step-by-step actions taken to meet a short-term goal or objective that can be part of a given strategy.
Blind date principle	When we accept as sufficiently complete information from a source that has incentives to share incomplete information so we will make the decision/act in the way that benefits them.
Fermi Method (Dimensional Analysis)	A multistep problem that can be solved in a variety of ways, and whose solution requires the estimation of key pieces of information.

Glossary

Law of diminishing returns	For the purposes of this book, the point at which the cost of information begins to exceed the benefit of its purpose.
Time series analysis (see also, trend analysis)	Process of comparing data over time to identify results or trends, which are then used to predict events and values beyond the end of the sequence.
Trend analysis (see also, time series analysis)	Process of comparing data over time to identify results or trends, which are then used to predict events and values beyond the end of the sequence.
Unbounded rationality	Decision-making that favors logic, analysis, evidence, and objectivity.
Uncertainty	A probabilistic problem in which the possible outcome (or outcomes) are measured in distributions.
Variable appraisal (see also, attribute appraisal)	In an attribute appraisal, we measure each event as a pass/fail. There is no gray area.
Vector	In mathematics, an object that has both a magnitude and a direction.

About the Author

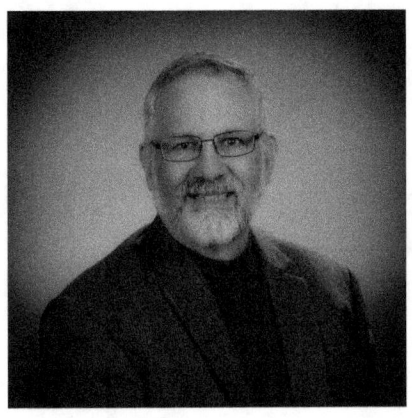

Frank Cohen

Frank Cohen is the Director of Analytics and Business Intelligence for Doctors Management.

Mr. Cohen is a computational mathematician with a focus on applied statistics, data mining, predictive analytics, and machine learning. The author of several books, including, "Lean Six Sigma for the Medical Practice" and "RVUs: Practical Applications for Medical Practices," Mr. Cohen has participated in and published numerous articles and studies and trained thousands of physicians, administrators, CPAs, and other healthcare professionals in all areas of healthcare analytics. His experience includes eight years as a Physician Assistant in both the Navy and as a civilian, clinic administrator and hospital CEO. His clients include hospitals, large and small medical practices, medical and professional associations, legal and accounting professionals, government agencies, and other healthcare professionals.

www.ingramcontent.com/pod-product-compliance
Lightning Source LLC
Chambersburg PA
CBHW052051220426
43663CB00012B/2529